The Art of Sensual Massage

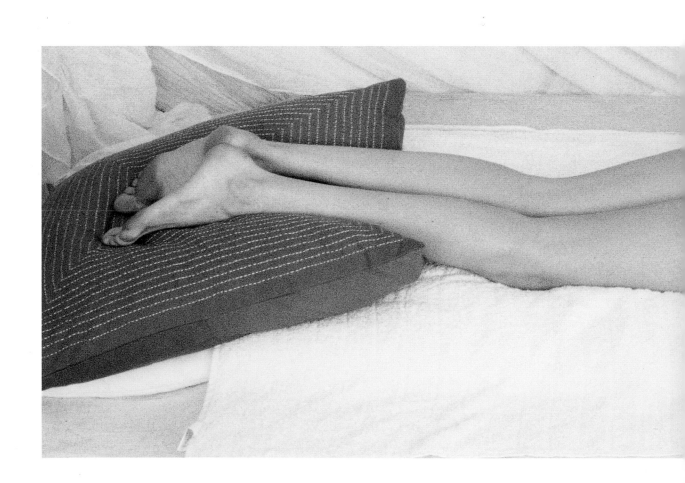

The Art of Sensual Massage

Marc Salnicki

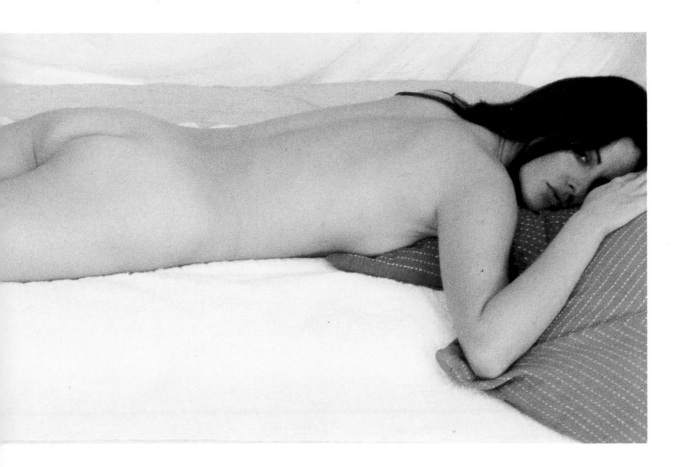

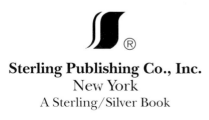

Sterling Publishing Co., Inc.
New York
A Sterling/Silver Book

A QUARTO BOOK

Published in 1999 by Sterling Publishing Co., Inc.
387 Park Avenue South
New York, NY 10016-8810

Distributed in Canada by Sterling Publishing
c/o Canadian Manda Group
One Atlantic Avenue, Suite 105
Toronto, Ontario, Canada M6K 3E7

Library of Congress Cataloging-in-Publication Data
Salnicki. Marcus.
    The art of sensual massage : techniques to awaken the
senses & pleasure your partner / Marcus Salnicki.
        p.   cm.
    Includes index.
    ISBN 1-4027-1369-X
    1. Massage.   2. Sensuality   3. Title
RA780.5.S25   1999
613.9'6--dc21   98-48689
                                            CIP

This book was designed and produced by
QUARTO PUBLISHING PLC
The Old Brewery
6 Blundell Street
London N7 9BH

PROJECT EDITOR Joyce Bentley
TEXT EDITORS Sarah Vickery and Nancy Terry
MANAGING ART EDITOR Francis Cawley
DESIGNER Caroline Grimshaw
PHOTOGRAPHER Will White
ART DIRECTOR Moira Clinch
QUAR.SNM

Manufactured by
Pica Colour Separation Overseas Pte Ltd, Singapore
Printed by
SNP Leefung Printing, China

This book is not intended as a substitute for the advice of a
health care professional or professional masseuse. If you have
any reason to believe you have a condition which affects your
health, you must seek professional advice. Consult a qualified
massage therapist, health care professional, aromatherapist or
your doctor before starting.

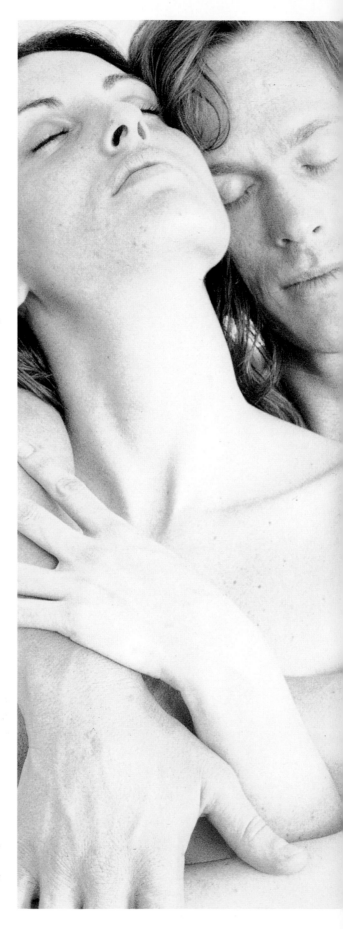

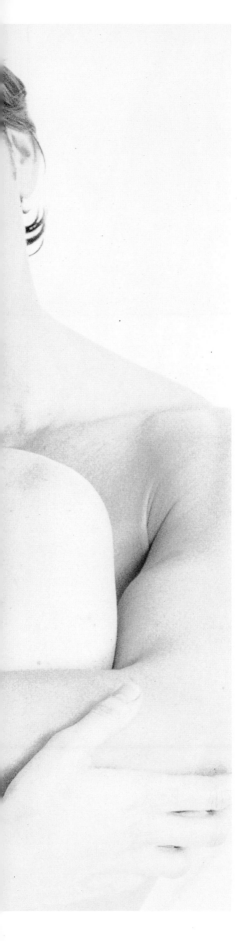

Contents

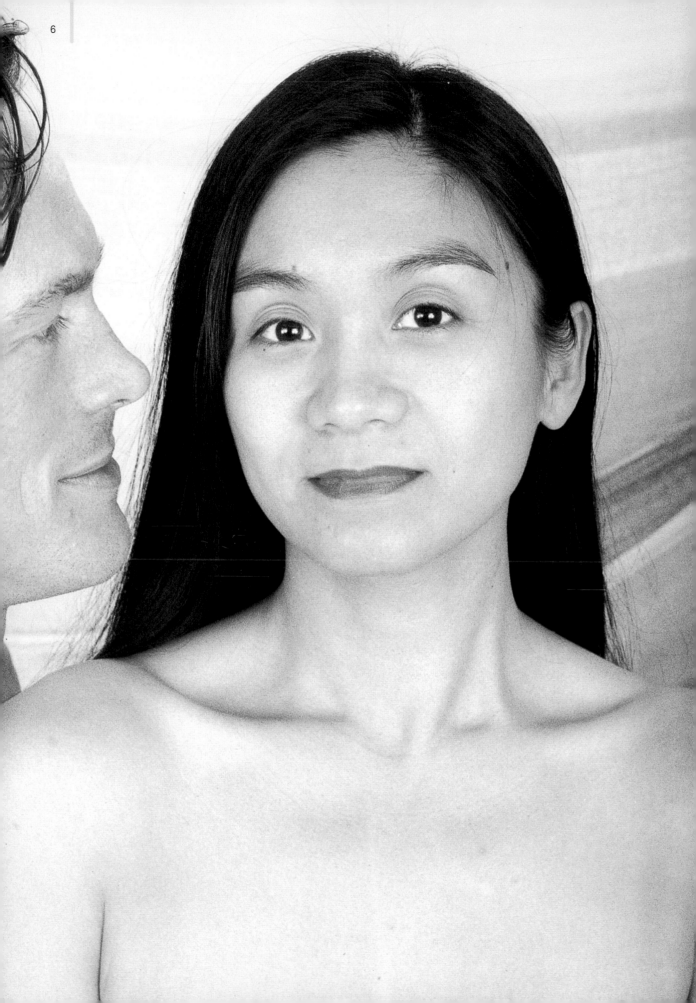

Introduction

The practice of massage has been handed down for centuries and its benefits are widespread. On a physical level it relieves aches and pains, regulates breathing, removes tension and restores flexibility in the muscles, breaks down waste products and cleanses the lymphatic system. On an emotional level a good massage is a relaxing experience, encouraging the release of endorphins, hormones which activate a feeling of well-being. When the body is relaxed it settles the mind and calms anxious emotions. Through massage both the body and mind is treated in unison. Relying on touch, massage uses several kinds of strokes to create different effects. For example the firm, circular

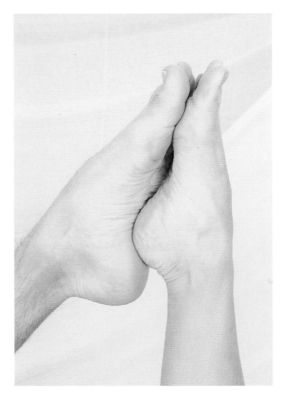

motion of the petrissage stroke is used around the muscle area to relieve tension and break down waste, while the gentle, sweeping movement of the effleurage stroke helps soothe and relax.

Sensuality in Massage

The sensual elements introduced in this book bring a more intimate level to the massage. In a relationship, massage is beneficial in enhancing the idea of touch and skin-to-skin contact. Sensuality is our ability to give and receive pleasure, requiring a full understanding of your partner's needs, and an appreciation of their responses. Combined with massage it creates a powerful expression of love.

Human contact is a necessary and healthy part of daily life, and one that if neglected can cause feelings of alienation within a relationship. From an early age parents can use massage to soothe a crying baby. It reinforces our sense of security and love, intrinsic to human nature. We rely on touch for emotional nourishment; to provide comfort, enhance intimacy, and encourage sharing. It is a form of communication that is based on intuition and understanding, rather than conversation. Its value is in helping to maintain a good relationship or to revitalize a tired one.

Everyday life can also add stress and pressure to a relationship, sometimes resulting in a breakdown of communication. Sensual massage is an unconditional way of removing that stress, and restoring harmony and balance. It helps us to learn about each other's bodies and desires, in a relaxed and loving environment. Sometimes sex can carry with it expectations of achievement and performance that may put pressure on one or both partners. The benefit of sensual massage is that it does not necessarily have to lead to intercourse. It is a reaffirming activity that can be enjoyed for itself, to induce sleep, or simply provide a forum for expressing emotion—it need only lead to intercourse if you so choose. Taking time to explore and understand each other's bodies is both exciting and fun. The beauty of sensual massage is that you do not have to be experts to enjoy it, as long as you are sensitive to your partner's responses and listen to their requests, paying particular attention to their pain threshold. It is the quality of the touch, and not the technique, that is important.

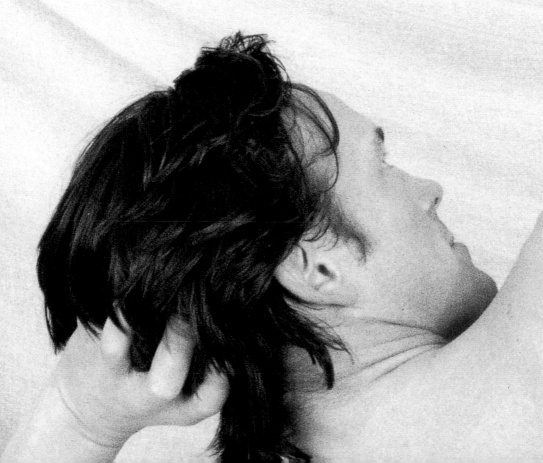

About this Book

In this book we take you on a journey of sensual massage, beginning with preparation. Some simple rules can make a massage a more fulfilling experience. Familiarizing yourself with massage procedures is both informative and enjoyable. Advice is given on the basics of giving and receiving a massage, and how to use the different parts of the body to full effect. You can even experiment with other stimuli, such as fabrics and feathers to enhance the overall effect.

An essential aspect of the massage is choosing the oil and learning how to apply it. Specific instructions are given for selecting your oils and warming the hands. An aromatherapy chart will help you select the oils most appropriate for the massage, and a recipe section gives you ideas for that special treat. Suggestions for setting the scene of the massage will help make it a more personal experience.

Basic Sensual Strokes will teach you the different types of strokes used in massage, and by practicing the techniques you can, in time, adapt them to suit your own preferences. The most common strokes are explained, and together they cover every aspect of massage. Some strokes work the tension out of muscles, with vibrant energizing strokes that awaken the skin, while the more gentle strokes induce relaxation. By working through the basic strokes you can perform a whole body massage or, if you have less time, choose to concentrate on the back or face.

As the central theme of a sensual massage is the exploration and understanding of your partner's body, a section on Massaging Your Partner focuses on the preferences of men and women. Discover your partner's erogenous zones, create a massage oil that will stimulate your partner's senses. You will see how a massage doesn't have to be restricted to the massage room but can be incorporated into everyday life. Experience the joy of shaving your partner, enjoying an invigorating shower together, or watching them relax while you wash their hair.

In Massage from Around the World you can draw inspiration from the traditional massage techniques of other cultures. In India massage is part of daily life, with skills passed down through generations. Use the techniques of the Indian chakra and mediation massage to explore hidden levels of communication. Japanese massage is renowned for its rituals of preparation as demonstrated in the foot massage. The Native American tradition used invigorating percussion strokes to re-energize the body, while the Egyptians favored bathing in sumptuous oils as a prelude to massage. As well as step-by-step massage instructions there are useful hints on how to transform your massage area to evoke the culture or region from where they came. Finally Sensual Treats explores the use of food in massage as an extra treat. It suggests ways you can use honey, cream or fruit to seduce your partner, and turn a celebration into a wonderful event.

After you have enjoyed the massage, experience the magical glow of warmth and satisfaction that it can create.

CHAPTER 1
The Language of Sensual Touch

In the art of sensual touch, the whole body can be used as a means of pleasure. Lightly dancing fingertips, strong forearms, caring, trusting hands, and a teasing tongue, all play a part in massage, and become powerful instruments of communication to relay feelings of desire and amorous pleasure.

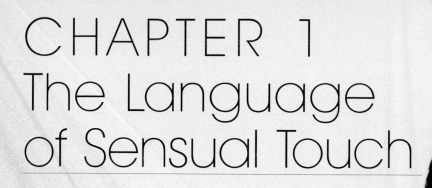

Skin-to-skin contact is probably the most intimate and erotic form of communication but there are endless other stimuli that can be used to complement massage or act as a form of foreplay, such as fabrics, feathers, hair or even ice cubes. All these will intensify your partner's feelings of sensuality. Imagine your partner lying naked on a soft, fragrant bed as you tease and tantalize their body to new heights of pleasure by dancing a peacock's feather over their skin. Now imagine it happening to you, and see how sparking your lover's imagination could lead to a higher level of intimacy in your relationship.

To enhance the experience of erotic massage and awaken your partner's sensual feelings, arouse their senses by burning seductive fragrances or incense before you massage them. Blend luxurious massage oils with aphrodisiac properties and savor the aroma. Ask your partner to close their eyes, and then tease their mouth with delicious sweet strawberries covered in honey, or the sharp zest of a grapefruit. Be adventurous with the build up to your massage and use items that will create a new sensory experience. This can also add an element of fun, giving you both a chance to relax before beginning the full massage.

Giving a Sensual Massage

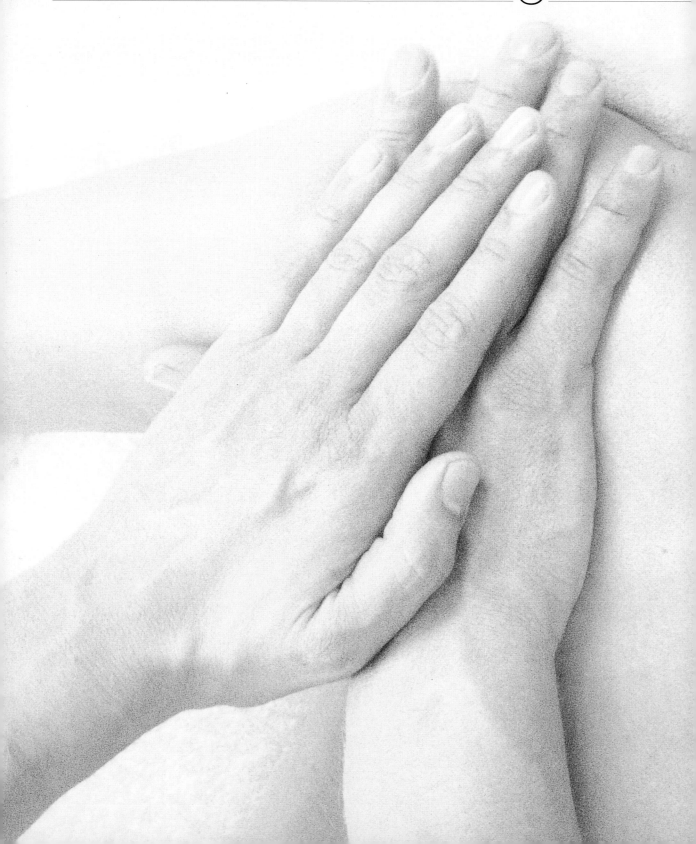

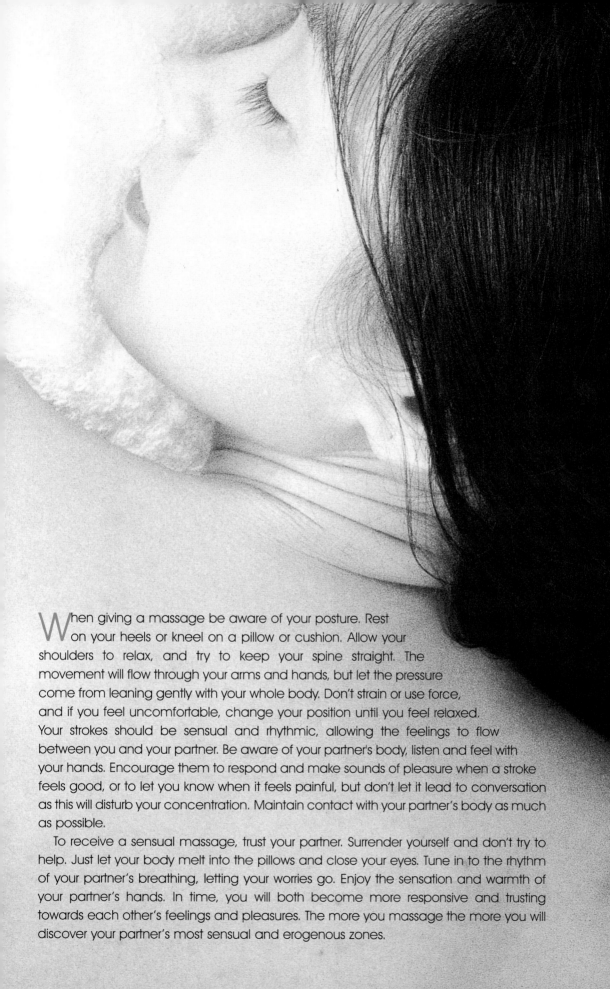

When giving a massage be aware of your posture. Rest on your heels or kneel on a pillow or cushion. Allow your shoulders to relax, and try to keep your spine straight. The movement will flow through your arms and hands, but let the pressure come from leaning gently with your whole body. Don't strain or use force, and if you feel uncomfortable, change your position until you feel relaxed. Your strokes should be sensual and rhythmic, allowing the feelings to flow between you and your partner. Be aware of your partner's body, listen and feel with your hands. Encourage them to respond and make sounds of pleasure when a stroke feels good, or to let you know when it feels painful, but don't let it lead to conversation as this will disturb your concentration. Maintain contact with your partner's body as much as possible.

To receive a sensual massage, trust your partner. Surrender yourself and don't try to help. Just let your body melt into the pillows and close your eyes. Tune in to the rhythm of your partner's breathing, letting your worries go. Enjoy the sensation and warmth of your partner's hands. In time, you will both become more responsive and trusting towards each other's feelings and pleasures. The more you massage the more you will discover your partner's most sensual and erogenous zones.

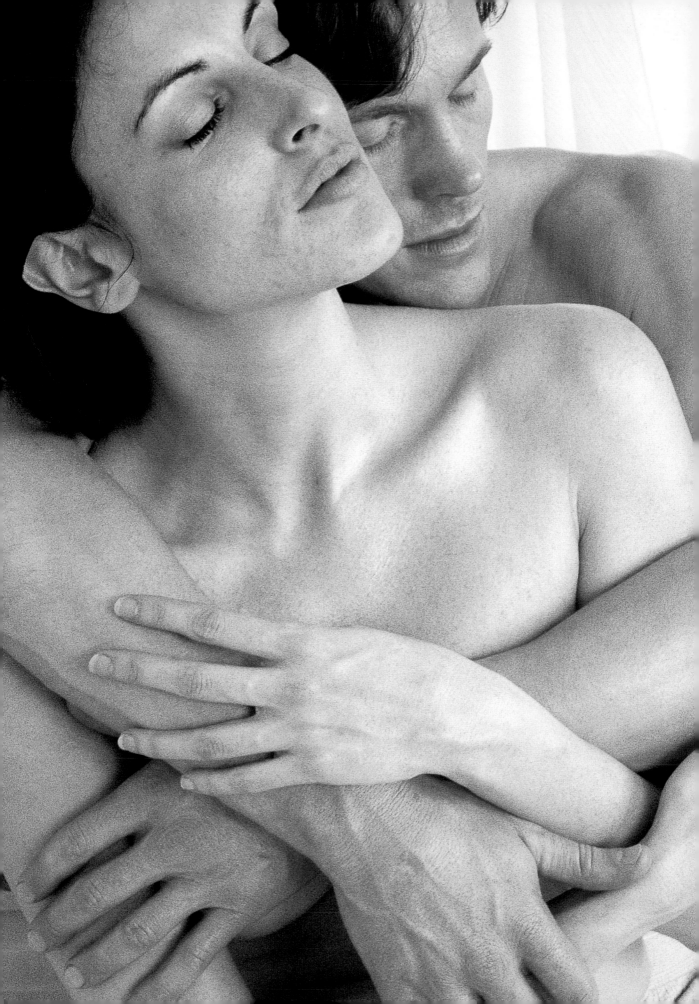

Caring Hands

A sensual caress, or a loving touch from someone's hands can sometimes say so much more than words. All too often we find it difficult to express our feelings to one another in a verbal way. Massage has a wonderfully powerful way of allowing us to express our feelings of love and trust through our hands. By gently and lovingly exploring your partner's body, and by caressing and stroking their most vulnerable areas, a special feeling of immense pleasure will flow between you, adding enchantment to your relationship.

As you begin to massage listen with your hands; respond to your partner's body when they move or sigh, and then linger in this area, using your hands lovingly to repeat the strokes they enjoy. Also become aware of their pain tolerance as their body

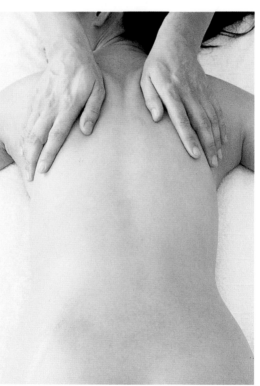

might be saying "it's time to move on" or "this stroke is too strong for me." Sensitivity is the key to ensuring complete fulfilment for your partner.

During massage your hands will become very powerful tools of pleasure as their movement across your partner's skin demonstrate your feelings. This is why it's so important that you look after your hands.

Before you start your massage, make sure they are clean and have no rough skin patches, and that your nails are short and smoothly rounded. Try warming your oil first by placing the bottle into a small bowl of hot water. If you suffer from cold hands, place a few drops of oil into your palm and rub your hands together prior to commencing the massage. Your partner will get pleasure from all the care you have taken with your hands.

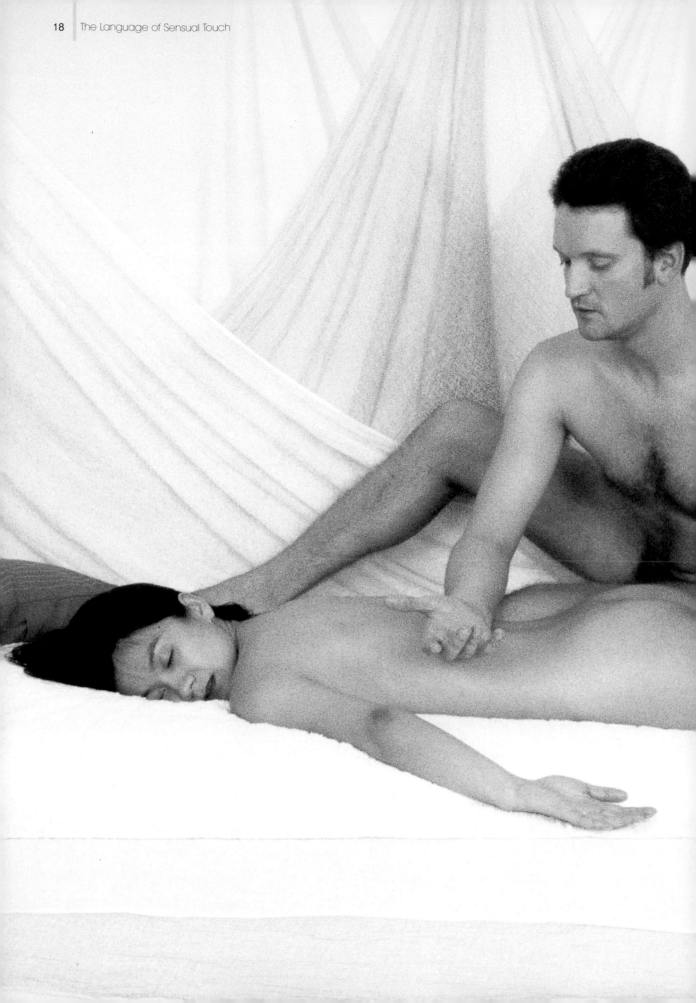

The Sensory Body

When using different parts of the body to massage be intuitive and experiment with your partner to discover their erogenous zones. Soft, clean hair has a divine, chiffon–like texture and can give wonderfully erotic sensations. If you have long hair, let it cascade over your partner's body, gently rocking your head from side to side to lightly tease the skin. Use your nails to set your partner's skin on fire by slowly teasing with long, shivering strokes. Then run your nails along the soft skin on the inside of your partner's arms, and along the length of the spine. Find the most sensitive areas of your partner's body, and then place a passionate, lingering kiss, or a long, slow lick of your tongue on their skin. Allow them to feel the soft, silky texture of your lips, or the hot, wet texture of your tongue. When you have moistened the skin, gently blow on it to create another nerve-tingling sensation. Caress the body with the forearms, especially the back and buttocks, and let the soft body hair send a shiver down the back. Alternatively, use the whole body for a different way of massaging. Cover yourself in oil and, lying on top of your partner's back, gently slide across the skin, nestling in the contours of their body.

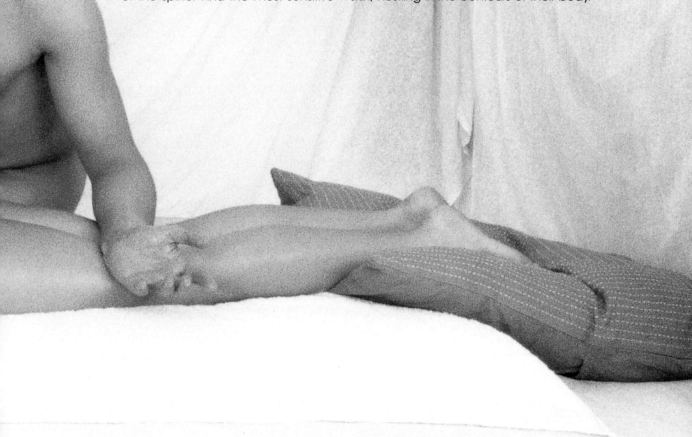

Sensual Stimuli

Reveal divine new pleasures for your partner by using objects to arouse different parts of the body. Caress and stroke them with soft, ticklish feathers or fine silk scarves. Experiment with different textures and sensations, to see how your partner responds to stimuli on different parts of the body. Torment and delight them by toying with the fabric, until the very pinnacle of desire is reached. You might also try drawing an ice cube over the skin and down the back, stimulating the nerve endings just beneath the skin. Tantalize your partner with the light-as-down touch of a baby-soft shaving brush, or the cold feel of a gold or silver necklace sliding over the skin.

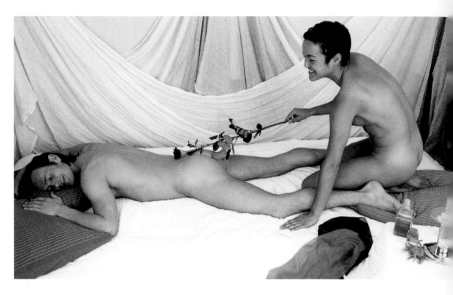

A Bouquet of Flowers

Choose a particular flower for its heady fragrance, texture, and color, or maybe because it is your partner's favorite. If you choose a rose, make sure the thorns are removed. Caress your partner's face with the flower head, allowing them to inhale the scent, then slowly run the flower over their body. Sprinkle some petals over the massage area, before using oils to complete the play.

The Sensation of Ice

Place an ice cube gently at the top of your partner's spine. Allow it to slide down the back, tingling the spine with it's cold sensations, and let it melt into the smooth curves of the lower back to experience the contrast between hot and cold. Gently massage the nipples with the cube and slide down toward your partner's navel.

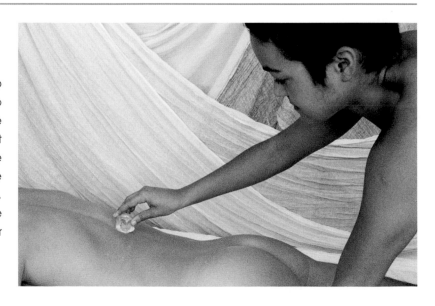

A Silken Caress

Use a beautiful silk scarf, a delicate piece of chiffon, or a rich, luxurious piece of velvet to slide slowly over your partner's skin. Allow it to caress each curve and muscle on your partner's body, as you use long flowing movements from the neck, down the back, over the buttocks, and down the legs. Softly tease the skin with the swaying movements of the fabric.

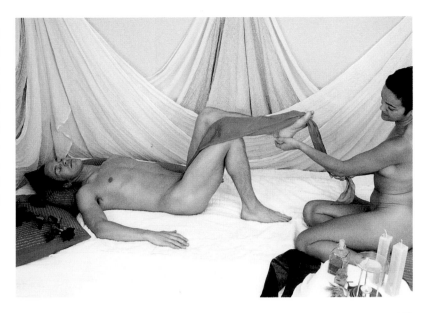

A Feather's Touch

Feathers are wonderfully sensual when brushed across the skin. Use a soft, clean one, or even a feather boa to caress your partner's body, slowly tickling and teasing their skin. Brush the inside of their elbow, which is extremely sensitive and erogenous, and caress the face and stomach. Spread the feather across the palms of their hands, before stroking it over their feet. Slowly draw the feather between each toe and tickle the feet to make them laugh.

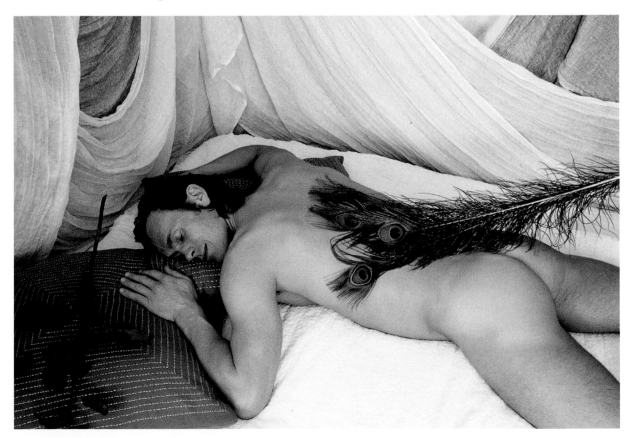

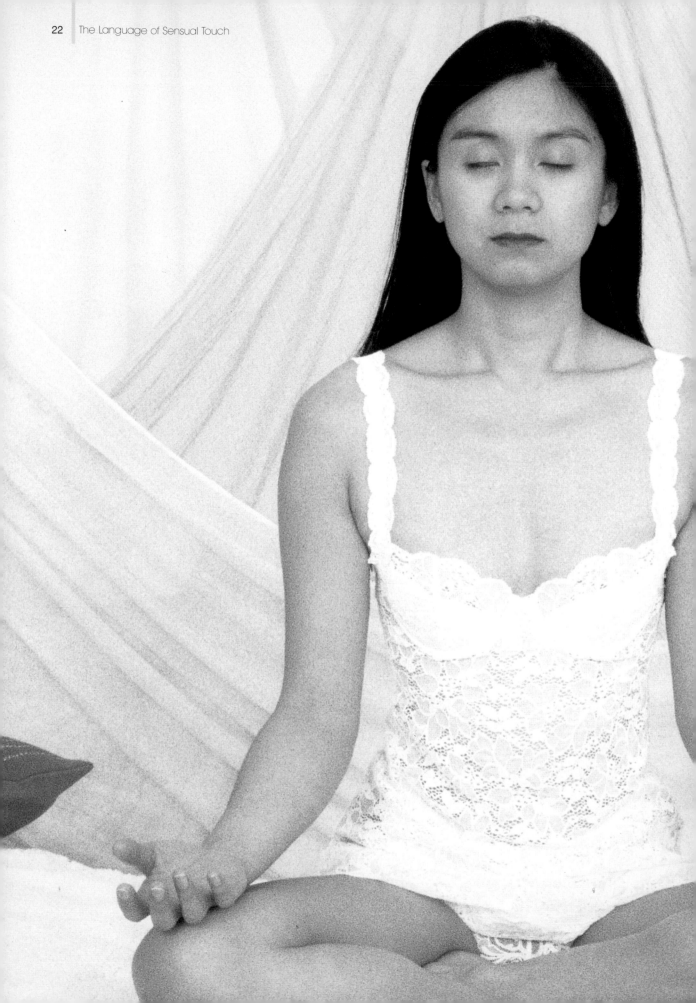

Preparing for Massage

Getting ready to give your massage should be an erotic process in itself—thoughtful preparation will be communicated through the massage. Mixing and blending delicious oils, grounding yourself mentally, setting the scene, warming your hands, and having everything ready for you and your partner is important and satisfying. Once you begin your massage, do not break contact with your partner or leave the room. Losing the skin-to-skin contact can spoil the whole ambience you have created, and break the sensual spell.

Creating a luxurious, warm room—filled with seductive fragrances and sensual massage oils—will help both you and your partner to relax and unwind. Be careful to choose both a time and a place for your massage that you and your partner will enjoy. Make sure

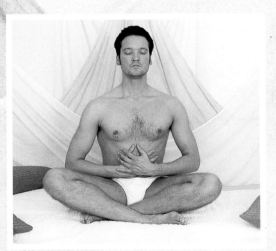

that you will not be disturbed, turn off the telephone and television, and do not answer the door. Try not to massage when you are tired, or only have limited time available, as the massage will be disappointing. It is better to relax and enjoy the massage when you are tranquil, have created a calm sanctuary, and have lots of time to explore your partner's body.

Once you have started seducing your partner with your sensual massage, and teasing their taste buds with chocolate-covered strawberries, you will have created a special bond between you. To keep this special feeling, try not to leave the room or break contact with your partner once you have started massaging. A way to prevent this is to make sure you have everything in the room that you will need, and to keep your massage oils within easy reach.

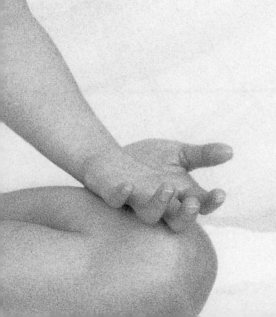

Warming the Hands

When performing your massage, keep your oil in a cork-topped bottle, or best of all, a plastic flip-top bottle. If you have nothing else to hand, use a bowl or a small jug, but be careful you don't knock it over. Your first application of oil to the hands should be done away from your partner so you don't spill oil on them. Pour a small amount into the palm of your hands and rub them together to warm and spread the oil. Then gently allow your hands to rest onto the body and start your stroke. To reapply the oil without breaking contact, turn one hand over and rest it on the body while pouring the oil with the other hand. Rub the oil between both hands and continue to spread the oil over your partner's body with broad, sweeping strokes. Reapply the oil as often as you need to keep your hands gliding over the body. Try not to over-oil the body, but also be aware of dry or hairy areas which may need extra oil.

Don't

Massage is contra-indicated with the following conditions:

- within two hours of eating a large meal
- flu or fever
- inflammation of skin or joints
- near open wounds, cuts or bruises, and bad skin conditions
- cancer
- during the first three months of pregnancy
- sprains or broken bones
- varicose veins and thrombosis

Do

- Respect your partner's requests
- Place all towels and oils within reach
- Maintain physical contact throughout
- Ask for feedback on your partner's preferences
- Keep the movements slow
- Prevent all conversation
- Create an uninterrupted environment

Preparing the Oils

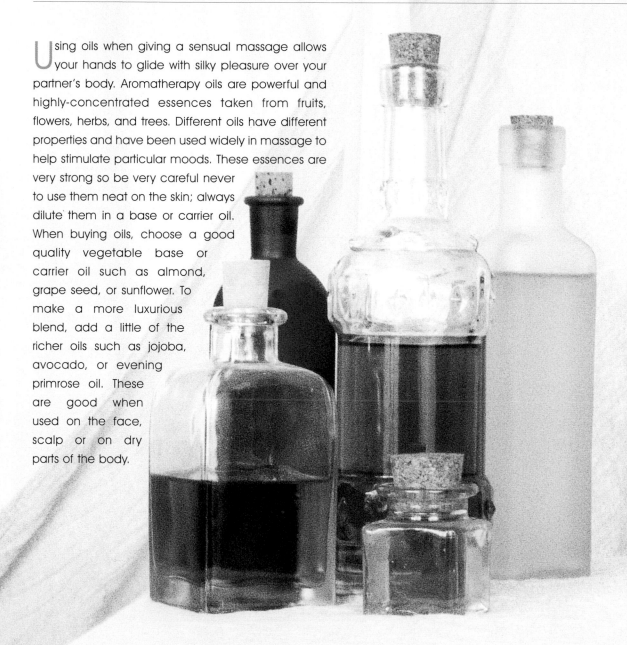

Using oils when giving a sensual massage allows your hands to glide with silky pleasure over your partner's body. Aromatherapy oils are powerful and highly-concentrated essences taken from fruits, flowers, herbs, and trees. Different oils have different properties and have been used widely in massage to help stimulate particular moods. These essences are very strong so be very careful never to use them neat on the skin; always dilute them in a base or carrier oil. When buying oils, choose a good quality vegetable base or carrier oil such as almond, grape seed, or sunflower. To make a more luxurious blend, add a little of the richer oils such as jojoba, avocado, or evening primrose oil. These are good when used on the face, scalp or on dry parts of the body.

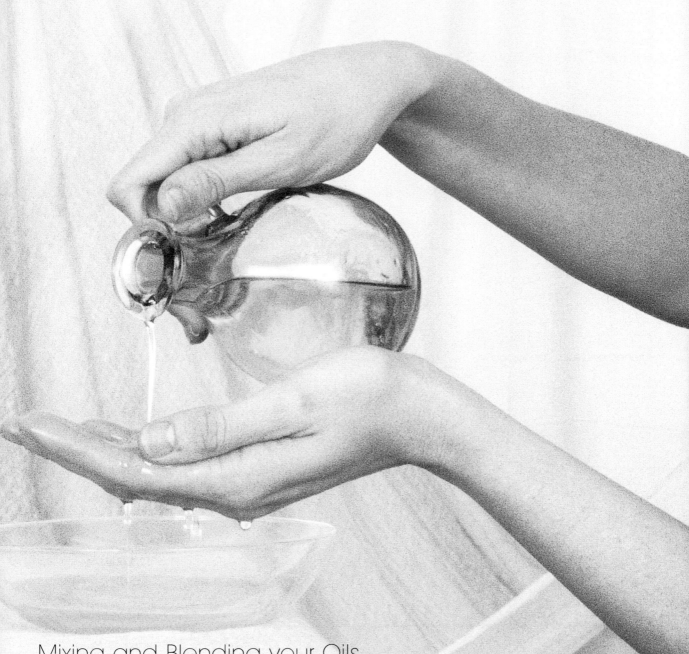

Mixing and Blending your Oils

You will need approximately 2 fl. oz. (50ml) of your base or carrier oil to massage a whole body. When making your own blend, bear in mind that aromatherapy oils lose their properties quite quickly once mixed with a base or carrier oil, so either use the mixture up, or add one teaspoon (5ml) of wheat germ oil to preserve their qualities. The Aromatherapy Chart provides a basic guide—these are just a few favorites but there are many more from which to choose. Blend sensual oils carefully to make sure they combine well with each other and do not clash. Subtlety is the key to successful seduction.

The Aromatherapy Chart

Oil	Therapeutic Use
BERGAMOT	stimulating: counters anxiety, colds, depression
CEDARWOOD	aphrodisiac: good for skin care, soothes respiratory disorders
CLARY SAGE	sensual, tonic: relieves stress, depression, nervous tension
FRANKINCENSE	calming: good for skin care, relieves stress and anxiety
GERANIUM	sedative: improves skin conditions, relieves depression and P.M.T.
JASMINE	mood enhancer: encourages well-being, relieves nervous exhaustion
LAVENDER	calming, healing: improves skin, relieves stress, insomnia, and muscular aches
LIME	tonic: relieves depression and colds
NEROLI (ORANGE BLOSSOM)	sedative, aphrodisiac: good for skin care, relieves depression
ROSE	healing, uplifting: improves skin, relieves depression and stress
SANDALWOOD	antidepressant, aphrodisiac: relieves stress, tension, and depression
SWEET ORANGE	uplifting: relieves depression and stress
VETIVER	relaxing: relieves insomnia, high blood pressure, and muscle pain
YLANG YLANG	relaxing: powerful aphrodisiac, relieves insomnia and stress

This chart shows some key essential oils and their characteristics, but many others are also available. Your local store will be happy to give you information about them.

Traditional Use	Warnings
a powerful, uplifting, refreshing oil named after the Italian city of Bergamot where it has been used for many centuries	do not use before sunbathing may irritate skin
this oil was used by the ancient Egyptians as a sacred burning oil and for cosmetic purposes	avoid during pregnancy
an aphrodisiac reputed to have a euphoric effect on the mind	do not use during pregnancy
a powerful aid to meditation, burned in ancient times as holy incense	
the flower is grown under the influence of the goddess Venus	may irritate sensitive skin
the beautiful scented flower is sacred to the Hindu god of love	may irritate sensitive skin
the Romans bathed in this for a feeling of calmness and peace	
inspires a feeling of happiness and well-being	do not use before sunbathing may irritate skin
an exquisitely fragranced oil used in bridal wreaths to help with nervous apprehension	
the queen of oils, a powerful feminine oil used by Cleopatra to seduce Marc Antony	avoid during early pregnancy
a warm, woody odor used in India and Egypt as a powerful aphrodisiac	
used when the spirit is low to uplift and cheer	do not use before sunbathing may irritate skin
the oil has been used in India for thousands of years as the oil of tranquillity	
in Indonesia, the flowers are scattered over the honeymoon bed to promote sensual desire and well-being	use in moderation—the fragrance is very powerful

Aromatherapy Recipes for Seduction

These recipes have been specially blended with luxurious base oils and rich aromotherapy oils to lavish on your partner. Choose exotic fragrances from around the world to enhance a massage or to tempt and tease your partner. Decide which mood you want to create and then mix the aromotherapy oils with 2 fl. oz. (50ml) of a base oil such as avocado, hazelnut, almond, or jojoba. Use on the body or in the bath, but for sensitive skin reduce the quanities by half.

Apollo

A masculine recipe for strength and sensuality

- 6 drops basil
- 4 drops frankincense
- 6 drops bergamot

Passion

To awaken and heighten the sense of desire

- 6 drops ginger
- 6 drops orange

Seduction

To allure your partner with the subtle scent of flowers

- 6 drops rose
- 4 drops ylang ylang
- 6 drops lemon

Shiva

To arouse the handsome Indian prince

- 8 drops sandalwood
- 5 drops patchouli
- 5 drops clary sage

Shakti

Specially prepared for a beautiful princess

- 6 drops geranium
- 4 drops patchouli
- 6 drops rose

Temptation

For an undeniably erotic moment of lust

- 6 drops cardamom
- 6 drops lime

Tranquillity

A calming blend for mind and body

- 8 drops lavender
- 5 drops clary sage
- 7 drops lemon

Venus

A potent combination of feminitiy and luxury

- 8 drops rosewood
- 4 drops ylang ylang
- 6 drops jasmine

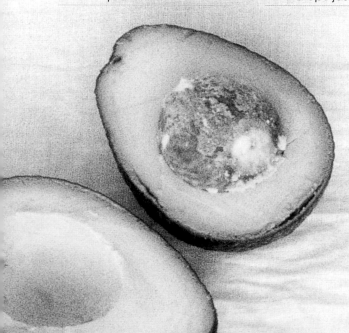
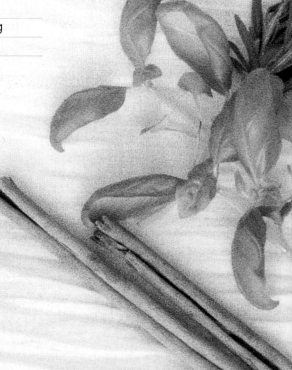

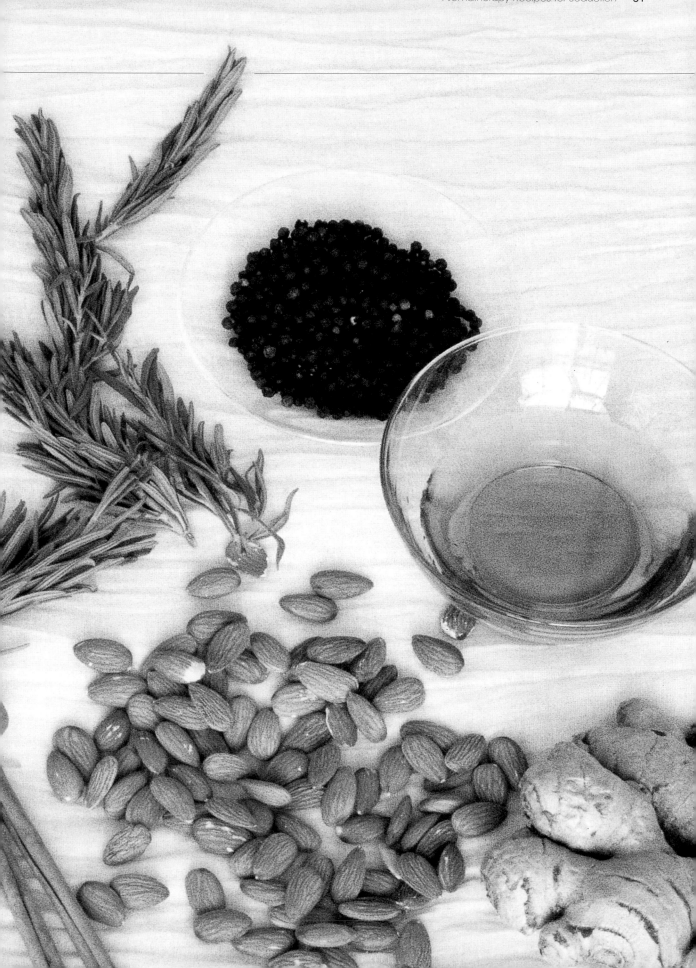

Setting the Scene

Creating your Sanctuary

Turn the room in which you are going to massage into a haven of pure pleasure, allowing your sensuality and fantasies to run wild. Fill the room with beautifully perfumed flowers, sumptuous exotic fruits, and deliciously tempting foods and wines to eat and drink. Create a seductive ambience by using the romantic light of candles, and playing soothing, sensual music to relax and calm you and your partner. Burn incense or exotic, sensual oils to fill the room with an exquisite fragrance. Use luxurious fabrics and sumptuous cushions to lie on. Your careful preparations will create a sensual environment in which to massage.

Lighting and Temperature

The room which your partner will step into should be as warm as a balmy, tropical night and bathed in a soft, seductive glow. Warmth is the most important ingredient when creating a comfortable setting in which to undress. It helps you to completely relax and surrender to your nakedness. Create seductive lighting using the warm, romantic glow of a flickering candle or nightlight. Place candle holders around the room for a special treat, and enjoy the soft glow of floating candles in a beautiful bowl, perhaps adding some of your favorite flowers or petals to the water. Try not to use the over-head lights, as they can be too bright; bring a lamp into your sanctuary if extra light is necessary. You could even change the light bulb to a soft, romantic colored one, to fill the room with a seductive glow.

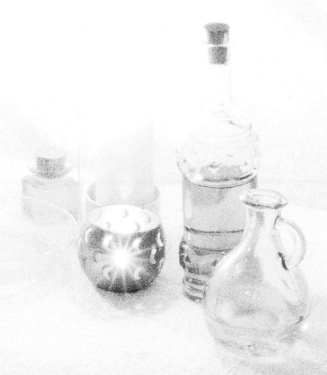

The Massage Surface

This area should be prepared with sumptuous, soft, warm fabrics and cushions. The floor is probably the best place to massage as it allows you to maintain contact with your partner, while still leaving room to move around. For the massage surface use a comforter, futon or blanket, and cover with towels or cotton sheets. An extra pillow under your own knees will allow you to be comfortable so that you can enjoy the experience with your partner. Above all, make sure you are both comfortable before you start.

Sound

The sense of hearing is particularly acute during massage as the ritual is usually carried out with the eyes closed. Before starting the massage eliminate as many distracting sounds as possible by switching off the phone, closing windows to street noises, and turning off appliances. Choosing music for your massage is a matter of taste, depending on the type of strokes you are using, but gentle music will enhance the mood of relaxation. Try the tranquil sounds of waves or dolphins, or perhaps some classical music would appeal. For the percussion massage you may prefer a more exhilarating drum beat, but whatever you choose make sure it is appropriate for the atmosphere.

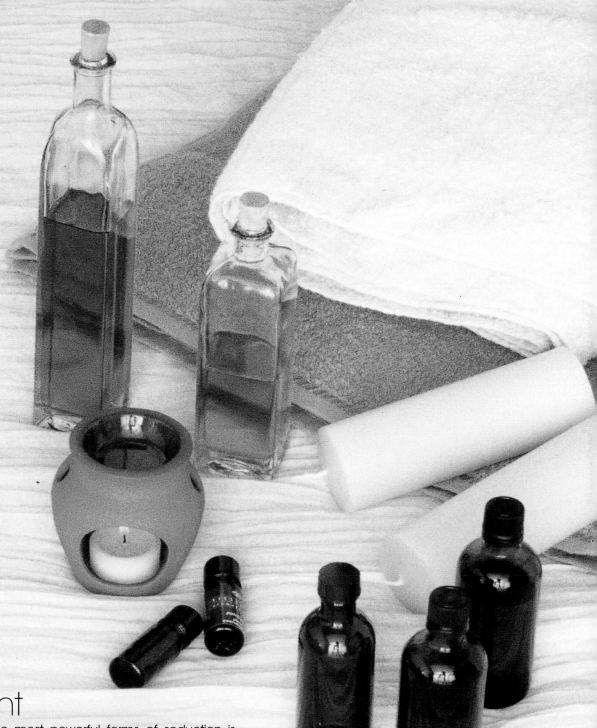

Scent

One of the most powerful forms of seduction is through the sense of smell. Being invited into a area that is filled with intoxicating fragrances such as rose, jasmine, sandalwood, or vetiver can be a wonderful way to start a massage. The burning of sensual oils, incense, or scented candles can also add a seductive enchantment to your surroundings. Choose one of your partner's favorite aromatherapy oils, sprinkle a few drops into an oil burner, and as the water is gently warmed it evaporates filling the room with an intoxicating fragrance. Alternatively, simply place a few drops on the massage bed or pillow.

CHAPTER 2
Basic Sensual Strokes

The following pages will show you the basic steps to giving a successful sensual massage. The strokes and routines we have created will enable you to do a wonderfully pleasurable, massage that is both fun and easy, and covers the whole body.

You may wish to delight your partner by incorporating some of the exotic strokes in the Massage from Around the World section, or tease them with the flickering, tickling strokes based on the more simple methods. You don't have to practice all the strokes, or even use them all the time. Sensual massage is about the pure joy of exploring your partner's body by using different strokes, ones that you know your partner loves, lingering on those that thrill them. The important thing is to just relax and enjoy yourself. It may take a little time to master the strokes or become comfortable with your partner, but the more you practice on each other, the easier and more erotic it becomes. You will soon start to discover your partner's most erogenous areas and follow the path of rapture together.

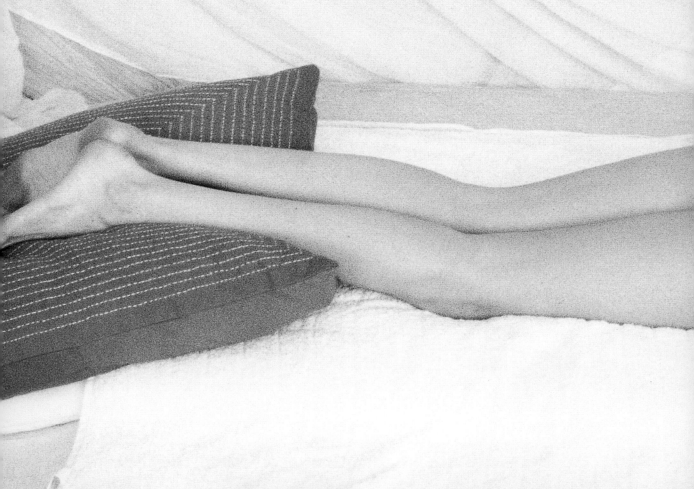

Our only recommendations are that you start your massage with the range of slow, rhythmic strokes that will spread the oil, relax your partner into the massage, and warm the muscles ready for the deeper strokes. Then complete the massage with light, caressing strokes to arouse your partner, letting them enjoy the tranquillity a massage brings.

The combination of relaxation, laughter, and stimulation will help you achieve greater intimacy in your relationship, and heighten your awareness of each other's needs, and the possibilities of each other's bodies. In Basic Sensual Strokes you will learn to master popular massage routines that you can practice and adapt to suit your preferences. You and your partner can then discover the joy of sharing sensual massage.

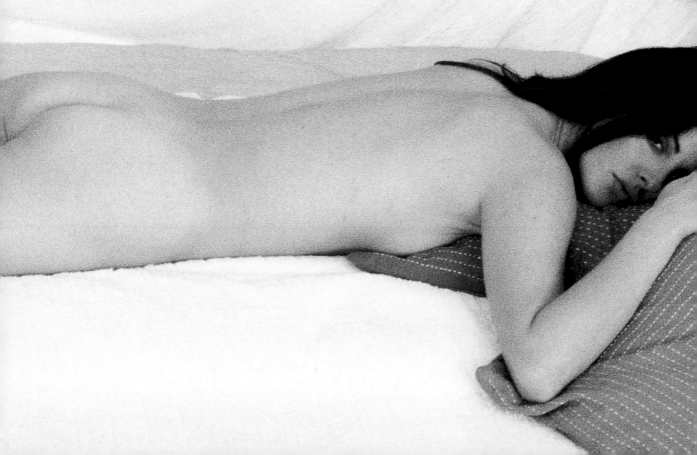

The First Touch

Now you have prepared the romantic and sensual scene and mixed your oils, it is time for that first magical touch. You may wish to bathe or shower together in warm, aromatic water before you start your massage. This will help you both to relax and unwind, and will awaken the skin.

Once you have invited your partner into your massage sanctuary, ask them to lie face down on the massage surface you have created. Make sure they are comfortable and warm, perhaps placing a pillow under the chest, pelvis, or knee areas for extra comfort. Once your partner has settled, kneel beside their lower back with your knees facing their head.

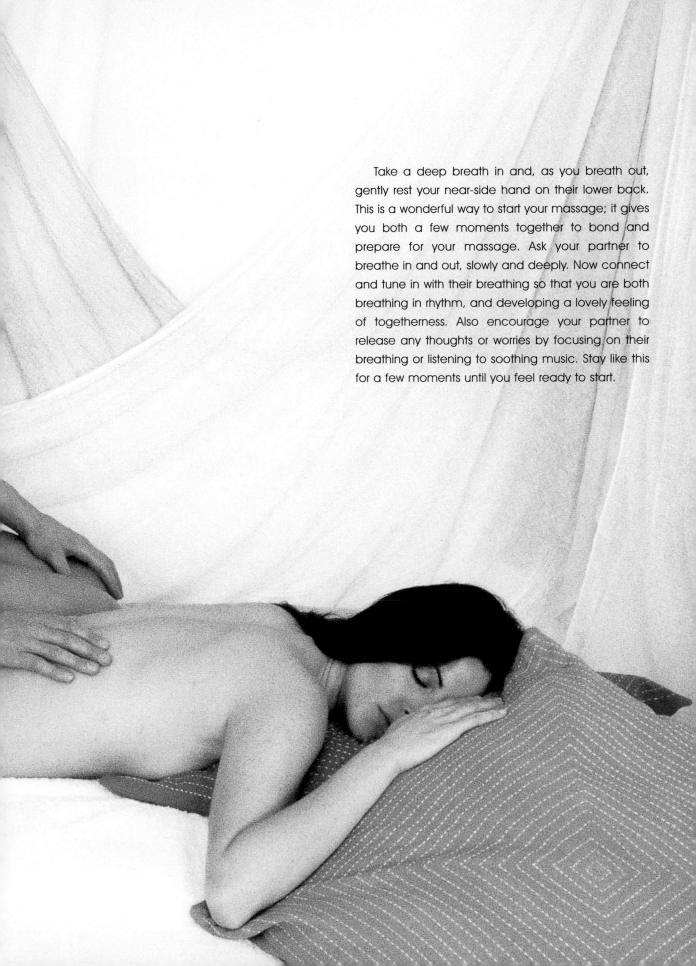

Take a deep breath in and, as you breath out, gently rest your near-side hand on their lower back. This is a wonderful way to start your massage; it gives you both a few moments together to bond and prepare for your massage. Ask your partner to breathe in and out, slowly and deeply. Now connect and tune in with their breathing so that you are both breathing in rhythm, and developing a lovely feeling of togetherness. Also encourage your partner to release any thoughts or worries by focusing on their breathing or listening to soothing music. Stay like this for a few moments until you feel ready to start.

Hand Positions on the Body

Effleurage

This soothing stroke is performed by using flat hands to apply an even pressure in a smooth, gliding motion. It is ideal for spreading the oil onto the body. It warms and relaxes the muscles in preparation for deeper work. Excellent for starting and finishing a massage, effleurage can be used all over the body. Apply deeper pressure toward the heart and less away from it to encourage the circulation of blood around the body, eliminating waste products via the lymph nodes.

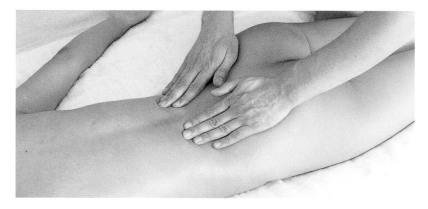

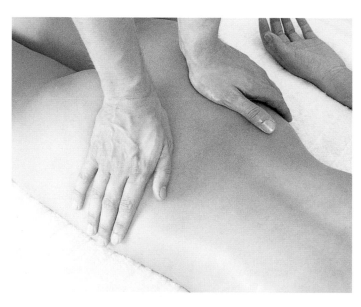

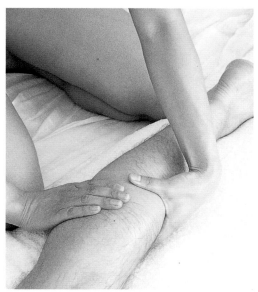

Wringing

Wringing is particularly useful on the calves and thighs. Use your hands to wrap around the leg with the thumb on one side and the index fingers on the other. With an even pressure, gently squeeze the legs, moving your hands in opposite directions. This literally wrings tension and stiffness out of the muscle.

Petrissage

A deeper massage stroke, using a firmer but slower pressure. Use the heels of the hands to apply pressure to muscles. Release to repeat the movement. Effective in breaking down waste products and releasing tension.

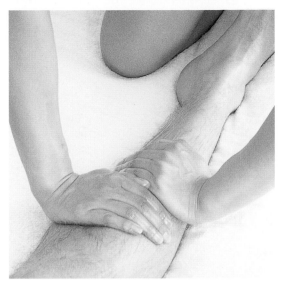

Cupped Hand Effleurage

This stroke is used mainly on the legs, molding hands in opposite directions around the calf. Use your outer hand to lead, as this allows your hands to turn easily over the top of the leg. Use light pressure moving downward as this will help to soothe, tired aching legs, and stimulate circulation.

Kneading

A deeper stroke used to squeeze waste and tension out of the muscles. It can be used on most parts of the body, especially fleshy areas. To massage imagine you are kneading a piece of dough then apply this theory to the body. Roll and squeeze the flesh maintaining a steady flow with both hands. Effective in manipulating the muscles.

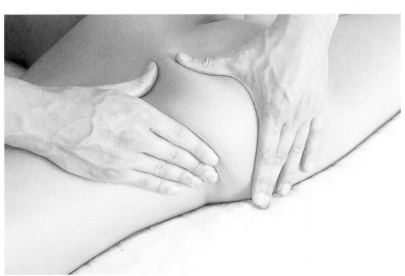

Percussion

A stimulating stroke used to energize the body and improve circulation. Your hands and wrists should be relaxed and loose then, using alternate hands, rapidly bounce the sides of your hands lightly on the skin in a series of brisk, rhythmic movements. Avoid being too heavy handed over the kidneys.

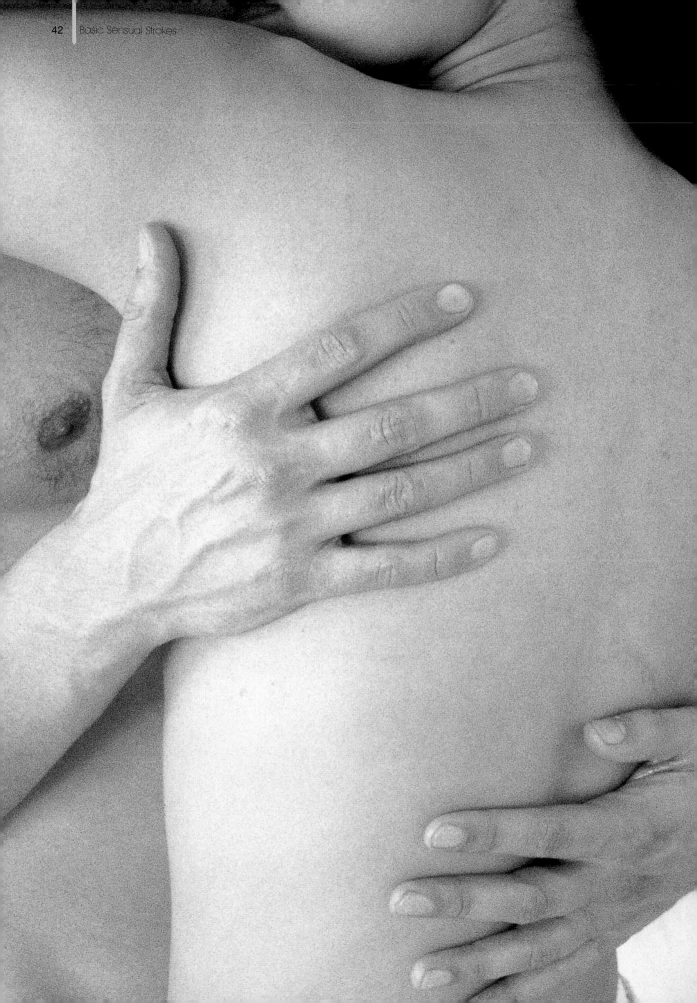

The Back of the Body

The back is a wonderfully sensual place to begin your massage as it has strong, powerful muscles to relax, and a myriad of nerves to tingle and bring alive, sending shivers of pleasure and delight through the whole body. The luxurious, broad surface of the back is ideal for your first strokes, and is also a less vulnerable area than some other parts of the body, allowing you both to relax into your massage and to build the confidence for other, more sensitive, areas of the body.

Effleurage on the Back

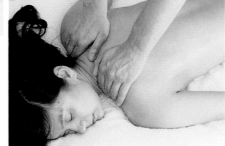

1 Sitting alongside your partner's lower back gently rest the warm palms of your hands on the curve of the lower back. With fingers pointing toward the shoulders, either side of the spine, slowly glide your hands up the back to the shoulders.

2 Allow your hands to slide over the top of the shoulders, gently molding them to the curves of the muscle.

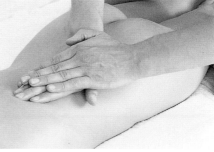

3 Slide your hands outwards to fan out across the top of the arms, shaping them to the contours of the body and sensually drawing them down to the back, to the starting position. Continue with this stroke several times.

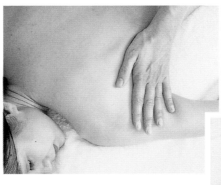

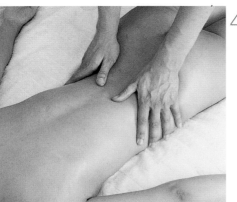

4 Place your hands on the top of the buttocks and slide them into the curve of the lower back. Slowly push your hands out to the sides and return them in a circular motion. Continue caressing up the back with circular strokes, before gliding your hands down the back, to the starting position. Repeat these strokes several times.

5 For the next stroke rest one hand on top of the other on the left-hand side of the lower back. Keeping your hands flat, glide them up and over the shoulders, drawing them out toward the arm.

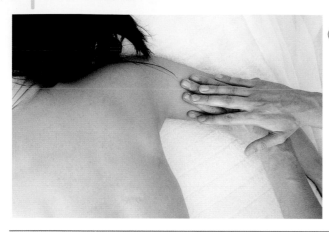

6 | Brush your fingers slowly down the arm, lingering on the hands before gently releasing. Move to the opposite side to repeat the stroke. You can do this several times.

Petrissage on the Back

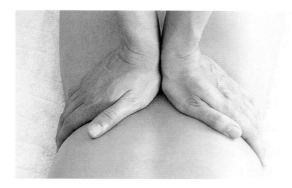 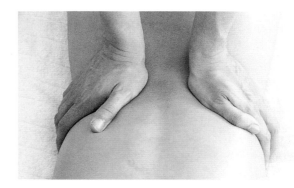

1 | Mold your hands over the lower back, the heels of your hands together either side of the spine and fingers pointing outwards. Gently lean on the heels of your hands and push them out toward the sides of the back.

2 | Keeping your fingers in the same position, release the heels of your hands, and then return to the starting position. Repeat this two or three times, gradually moving up the back to just below the shoulder blades. Glide your hands down the back to the starting position and repeat.

Kneading

1 | Rest your partner's arms above their head. Kneel facing your partner's back with your knees apart. Place your hands on the opposite side of your partner's back, thumbs away from your fingers.

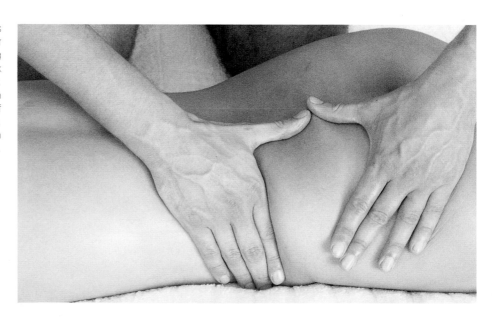

2 Glide one hand up the sides of the back, gather up the flesh, squeeze it, and then release it into the opposite hand. Continue this movement up and down the whole side of the back and buttocks. Move to the opposite side to repeat the stroke.

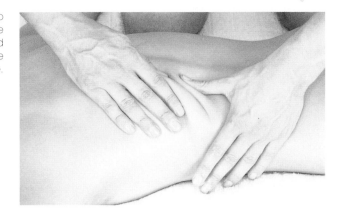

Petrissage on the Shoulders

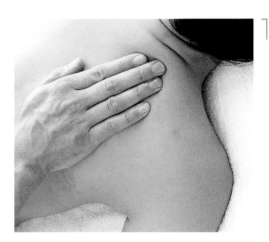

1 Kneel beside your partner's upper back with their head turned away from you. Place one hand flat on the upper shoulder, the other just below.

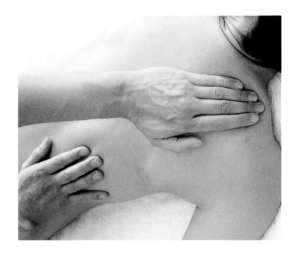

2 Keeping your hand flat, apply pressure with the heel of your hand. Push up toward the shoulder, and mold your hand over the front of the shoulder. Relax the pressure and pull your hand back. Repeat these strokes sliding alternate hands past each other.

The Back of the Neck

1 Ask your partner to rest their forehead on the backs of their hands. Rest one hand on the back of the head to keep it steady, while the other gently but firmly squeezes the base of the neck. Work slowly up the neck, squeezing and releasing in a circular motion. Now work back down the neck. Return to your partner's side and ask them to rest their arms back down by their sides and finish with effleurage.

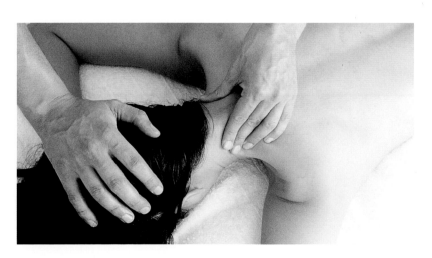

The Legs and Buttocks

The back of the legs and buttocks, with their erotic curves and creases, make them a very sensual area to massage. Stroking and kneading the soft, fleshy, round buttocks can create feelings of arousal. There is nothing more relaxing than the ecstasy of having someone massage the legs to improve circulation, and ease tired muscles, or just simply to caress and adore them. When massaging the legs, relax the pressure over the backs of the knees and use plenty of oil on hairy legs.

Back of Leg Effleurage

1 | Sit astride your partner's foot or kneel beside it. Place your hands flat on the lower leg just above the ankle, with your index fingers together. Slowly glide your hands up the leg, caressing the contours of the muscles, and moving your hands to the top of the buttocks.

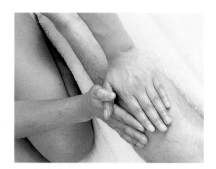

2 | Slightly separate your hands and your fingers and draw them slowly and lingeringly down each side of the leg. Repeat the stroke several times.

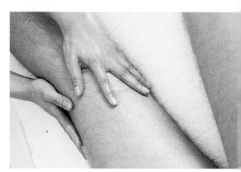

3 | Mold your hands in a cupped position on the lower calf. With your fingers pointing in opposite directions, gently lean on them. Keep your hands in this position and move them up the leg toward the buttock.

Wringing

1 | Change your position so you now face your partner's calf. Wrap your hands around the calf muscle on opposite sides, with your thumbs away from your fingers. Squeeze the muscle, and gently glide your hands past each other so when one hand is pushing the other is pulling.

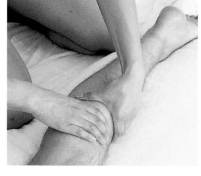

2 | To work the thigh, position yourself near the thigh and move your hands up the leg. Repeat the wringing stroke, but this time place your thumbs next to your fingers to squeeze and lift the thigh as you wring.

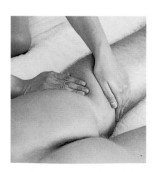

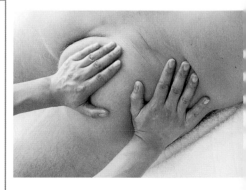

4 | Slowly open and fan out your hands and fingers to each side of the buttock, and draw them down the leg.

Pettrisage on the Leg

1 | Sitting astride your partner's leg, place both hands on the lower calf with the heels of your hands together, and your fingers pointing away from each other. Gently lean onto the heels of your hands, pushing them apart in an outward direction, and then release the pressure. Repeat the stroke as you move slowly up and down the calf.

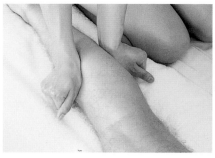

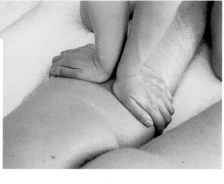

2 | Sit astride your partner's calf and repeat the petrissage stroke, starting just above the knee and ending just below the buttock. Continue this stroke slowly up and down the thigh.

Effleurage on the Buttocks

1 | Sit astride your partner's thighs and place your hands on your partner's buttocks in a diagonal position, with your fingers facing the same way. Push and slide over the mound of the buttock. Keep your hands flat and mold them into the curve of the lower back.

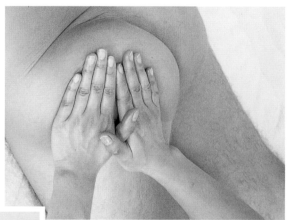

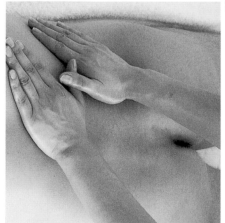

3 | Cross over your partner's body and kneel beside your partner's legs, facing their buttocks. Rest both hands on the opposite buttock. Lean in with the heel of one hand, keeping the hand flat, and glide down the side of the buttock. Pull back up with a flat hand, and repeat the stroke with the other so that the hands cross over.

2 | Separate your hands and draw your fingers round the buttocks, back to the starting position. Repeat this stroke several times.

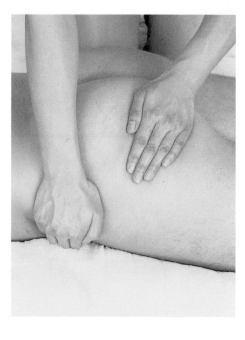

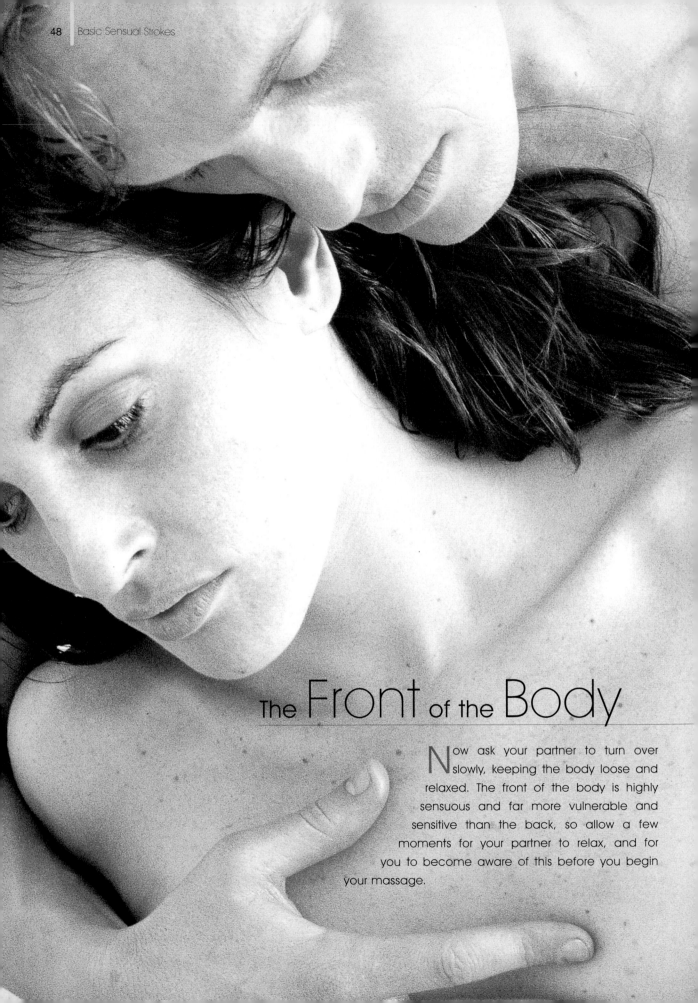

The Front of the Body

Now ask your partner to turn over slowly, keeping the body loose and relaxed. The front of the body is highly sensuous and far more vulnerable and sensitive than the back, so allow a few moments for your partner to relax, and for you to become aware of this before you begin your massage.

The Chest and Neck

The chest is a deliciously erotic area, for both men and women. By using caressing, sweeping strokes across the chest, you can create a divine feeling of openness, love, and abandonment as the chest and lungs heat up and react to caring hands. To heighten the sensations further, there are the sensitive nipples to arouse through tantalizing touches.

The neck is often very tense and stiff, causing problems throughout the whole upper body. Caressing, squeezing, and kissing the neck will allow your partner's muscles to melt in your loving hands, causing the upper body to feel an amazing sense of release and calm.

Effleurage on the Chest

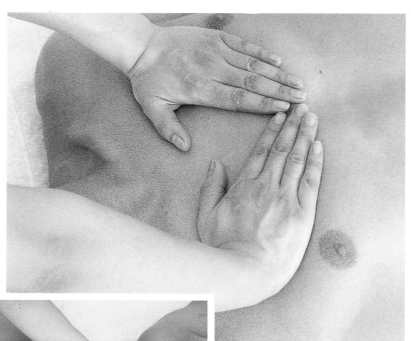

1 | Kneel astride your partner's head, and gently place your hands on the chest, with your fingers facing each other. Maintain this position for a few moments as you breathe deeply and evenly. Slowly separate your hands, and glide them over the front of the chest toward the shoulders.

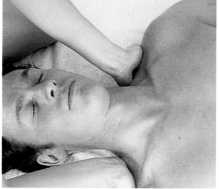

2 | Mold your hands over the top of the shoulders, bringing them beneath the shoulder.

3 | Push the shoulders lightly toward the feet before drawing your hands along to the neck. Turn your fingers in around the neck and draw them underneath the back of the neck to the scalp and off the top of the head. Repeat this stroke several times.

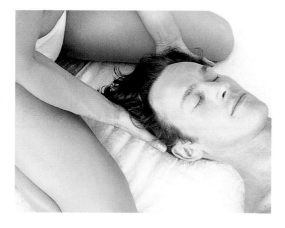

Squeezing the Neck

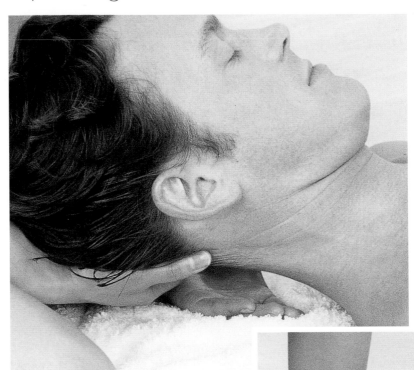

1 | Place one hand beneath the back of the neck, just above the shoulders. Cup your hand and squeeze the neck, slowly drawing your hand up the neck to the base of the skull.

2 | Repeat with the other hand before the first hand has fully lifted away from the neck. Keep repeating this stroke to achieve a flowing movement with both hands.

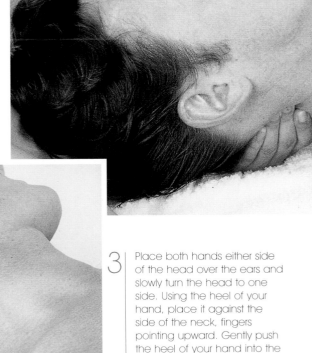

3 | Place both hands either side of the head over the ears and slowly turn the head to one side. Using the heel of your hand, place it against the side of the neck, fingers pointing upward. Gently push the heel of your hand into the neck and glide it down the neck to the shoulder. Repeat on both sides of the head.

Squeezing the Chest

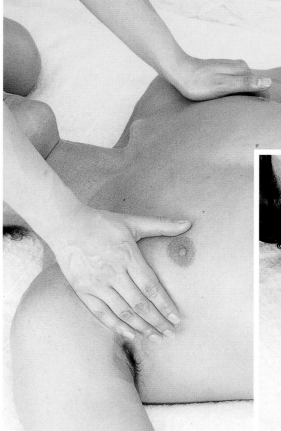

1 Place the heels of the hands on the chest muscles, fingers facing outward. Move your hands to the breast area.

2 With your thumbs facing inward curl your fingers lightly under the muscle just above the armpit, with the flesh of the breast area between your fingers. Push down on the muscle, moving the heel of the hand outward. Repeat on both sides.

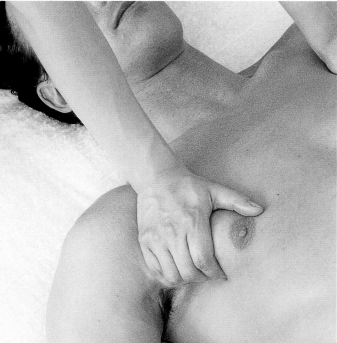

3 Complete with effleurage strokes, place your hands together on the breastbone, drawing them up toward you and then out toward the shoulders.

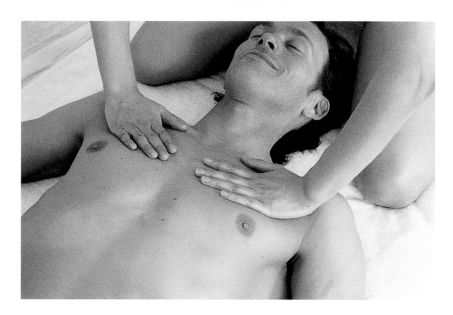

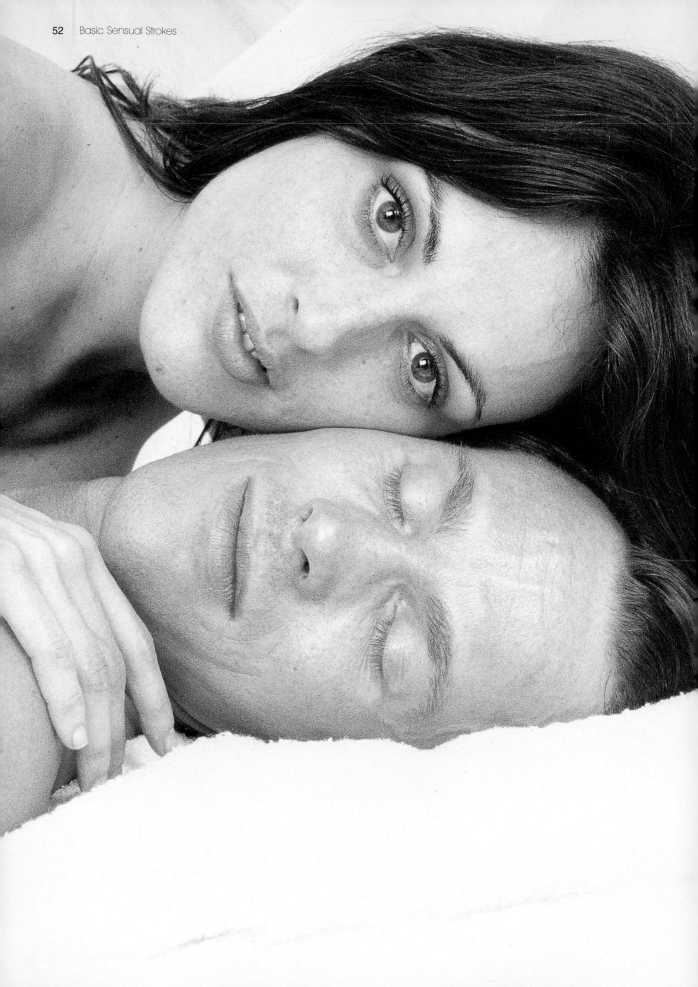

The Face

The face is one of the most sensitive and delicate areas of the body, full of sensuality with soft, kissable lips, adoring eyes, and angled cheekbones all crying out to be touched and caressed. Not until we receive a face massage do we realize just how much stress it bears. As slow, gentle, loving hands start to work across the face, vitality is restored and stress dissolves away, leaving a feeling of tranquillity and a blissful calm that will seep through the whole body.

Forehead

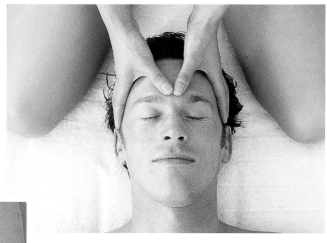

1 | Kneeling astride your partner's head and using only a small amount of oil, gently and slowly mold your hands over your partner's forehead, thumbs resting in the center just above the eyebrows. Stay in this position for a few moments so your partner becomes accustomed to your hands.

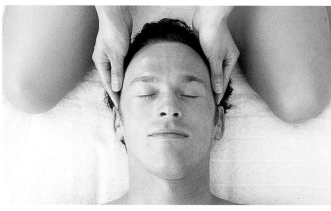

2 | Using the pads of your thumbs, firmly but gently slide them out toward the hairline, and lift your hands away and repeat.

3 | Gradually start to work up the forehead, one stroke slightly above the other, until you reach the hairline. Then slowly work back down the forehead to the eyebrows.

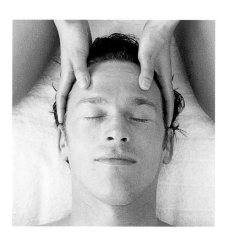

Eyebrows

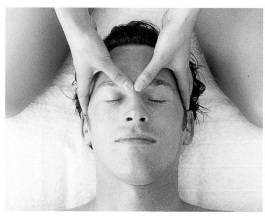

1 | Rest the pads of your thumbs just above the bridge of the nose, level with the eyebrows.

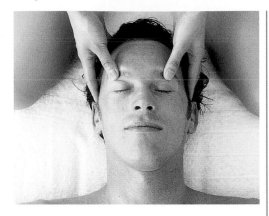

2 | Glide your thumbs across the eyebrows until you reach the hairline, being careful not to drag the skin around the eyelid. Lift your thumbs off, and repeat the stroke.

Temples

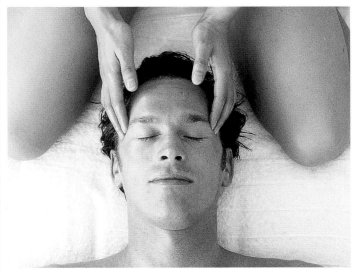

1 | Kneel astride your partner's head and, using the soft pads of your fingers, gently rest them on your partner's temples and massage them with slow circles.

Cheekbones and Ears

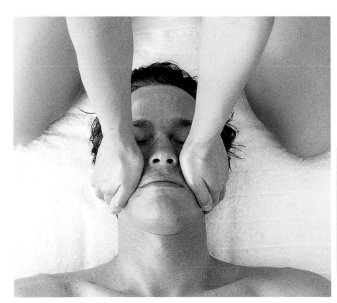

2 | Slide the heels of your hands over the cheekbones and down over the ears. Squeeze the ears with your fingers as the hand slides off, leaving the fingers where they are. Repeat the strokes with the heel of your hand.

1 | Place the heels of your hands on your partner's cheekbones, hands wrapped around the face and fingers beneath the ears.

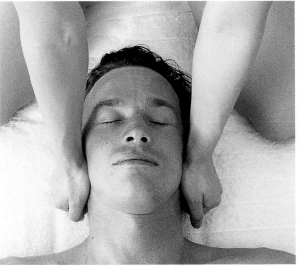

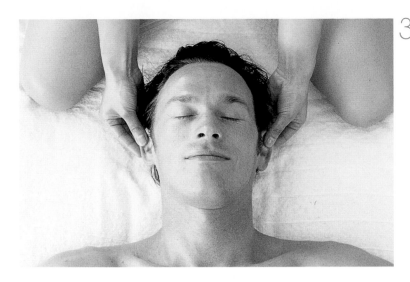

3 | The ears are an astonishingly erotic area and worth indulging with a little time. Massage them slowly and sensuously using the pads of your index finger and thumb. Gently squeeze the earlobe with firm, slow movements and massage the outer ear with small circles before returning to the ear lobe. Work over the ear three or four times.

Jaw and Lips

1 | Use the pads of your fingers to gently massage the cheekbone and jaw. Start near the nose and slowly work out toward the ear using firm, small circles. Repeat by coming back in toward the nose.

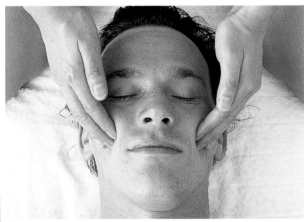

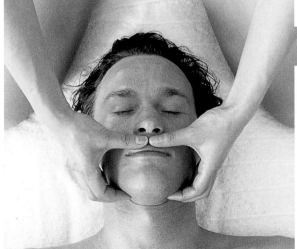

2 | Gently rest the pads of your thumbs pointing inward on the area between the nose and upper lip. Slowly slide your thumbs out toward the corners of the mouth. Gently lift away your thumbs, and repeat the stroke from the beginning three or four times.

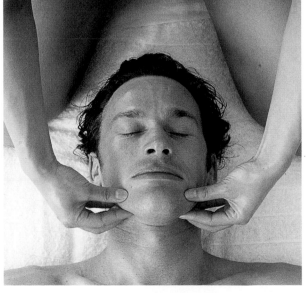

3 | Repeat the stroke, but this time gently place the pads of your thumbs between the lower lip and jaw before sliding them out to the corners of the mouth.

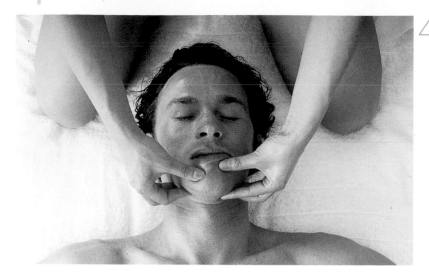

4 | Hook your fingers beneath the jaw, and gently squeeze the jaw and chin while slowly rotating your thumbs in alternate circles on the chin. Separate your hands, while still rotating, and squeeze the jaw. Work out toward the ears, lifting your hands away to repeat the stroke.

Chin to Forehead Effleurage

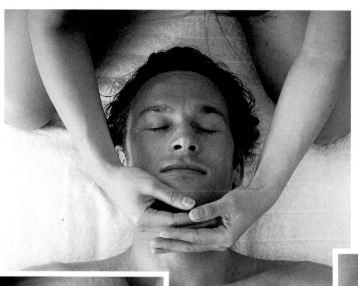

1 | Cup your hands around the chin. With your hands flat, slowly draw them up either side of the face, gently pulling as you go.

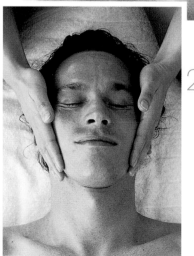

2 | Allow your hands to caress your partner's face as they draw up toward the forehead.

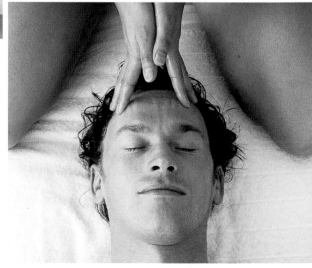

3 | Finish the stroke with the fingertips gliding across the forehead.

4 For the next stage of the massage use the fingertips, drawing them across the chest and then up either side of the neck.

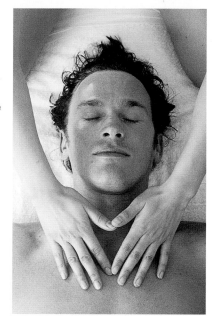

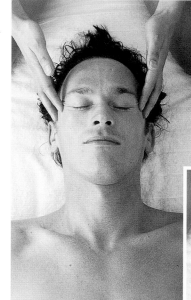

5 Gently draw the pads of your fingers up the sides of the face, over the forehead and into the hair in one long, sweeping stroke.

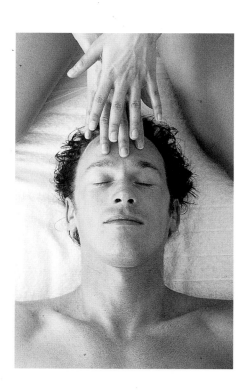

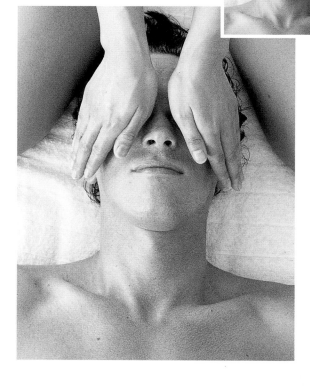

6 Continue with your fingers wide apart, and use just the tips to brush over the forehead from the brow to the hairline. Follow one hand after the other, and gently move from left to right, brushing the whole forehead.

7 To complete your face massage, rub your hands together to create some warmth and then, very gently, rest the palms of your hands over your partner's eyes. This will block out the light giving the eyes a complete rest. Maintain this position for a few moments, closing your own eyes too. Wish your partner some wonderful, loving thoughts and imagine these thoughts rolling down your arms and hands into your partner. Lift your hands away slowly. Then gently lean over, and kiss your partner on the lips.

The Arms and Hands

Arms and hands love to be held and touched, especially the soft palm of the hand as it is so sensitive. We use our arms and hands in so many different ways to express our feelings of joy, love, and anger both at work and at play. Overuse is often made of them, and tiredness and fatigue creep in; massage is a wonderful way of allowing life and energy to flow back through them. Using your hands to massage the hands of a loved one can strengthen a loving relationship. Caressing your partner's hands, entwining fingers together, and seductively kissing each finger in turn will send them into pure heaven.

Effleurage on the Arm

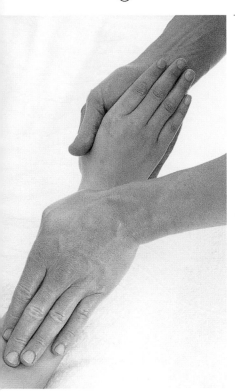

1 | Kneel beside your partner's arm. Hold your partner's hand, with his or her palm in yours and rest their elbow on the floor. Place your other hand on your partner's wrist, fingers pointing toward the shoulder, and slowly glide up the arm to the shoulder, spreading your fingers apart and slowly caressing the arm before sliding down the outer arm. Repeat the movement several times.

Cupped Hand Effleurage

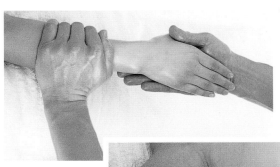

1 | Place one hand in a cupped position, and wrap your fingers over the wrist. Glide the hand up the arm to the shoulder, keeping a steady pressure as your fingers open out.

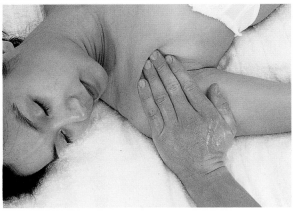

2 | Curve your hand around the shoulder, and draw your fingers back down the arm. Repeat this stroke several times creating a wonderful, flowing stroke.

Kneading

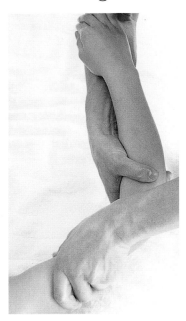

1 | With one hand, hold your partner's elbow and lift the arm off the floor. Rest your partner's hand on your elbow. With your free hand, thumb one side of the arm, fingers on the other, gently but firmly squeeze the whole upper arm.

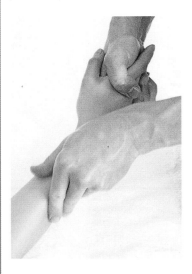

2 | Lower the arm and lift the forearm off the floor. Hold your partner's hand and gently squeeze the forearm with your free hand.

Petrissage on the Hands

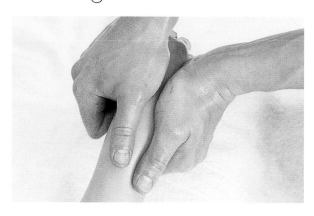

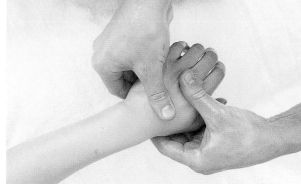

1 | Take your partner's arm and pick up their hand. Place the heel of your hands on the back of theirs, wrapping your fingers around the palm. Spread the heels out across the back of their hand and knuckles, then return to the starting position. Repeat this stroke several times.

2 | Keep your fingers in the same position and rotate the pads of your thumbs in small circles over the back of the hand.

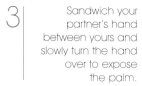

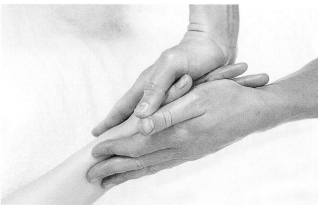

3 | Sandwich your partner's hand between yours and slowly turn the hand over to expose the palm.

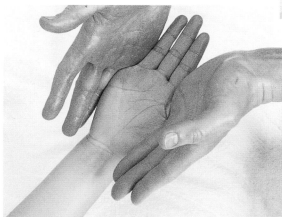

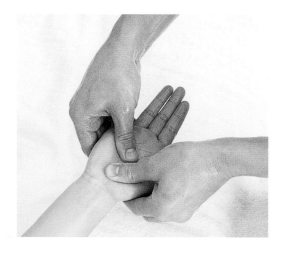

4 | Hold your hands out, palms up, and spread your fingers. Ask your partner to slide their hand between your little and third fingers so that their thumb and little finger protrude on either side.

5 | From this position use the pads of your thumbs to make slow, firm circular motions across the whole of the palm and wrist area.

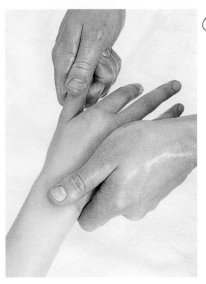

6 | Turn your partner's hand over, palm down, and hold it. Take their little finger at the base, and use your thumb and index finger to gently squeeze and rotate it. Pull and caress until you reach the fingertip. Repeat the stroke on each finger.

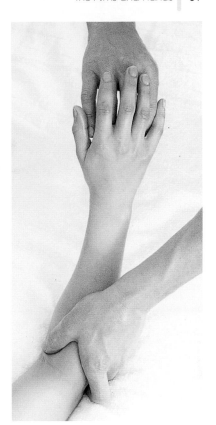

7 | Hold your partner's forearm with one hand and glide the back of your other hand slowly beneath theirs until you reach the end of hand.

8 | Entwine your fingers into theirs, Squeeze your fingers and slowly slide them through, pulling gently as you work your way to the end. Repeat this stroke several times.

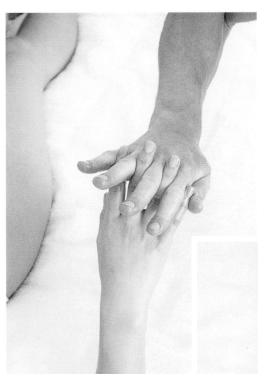

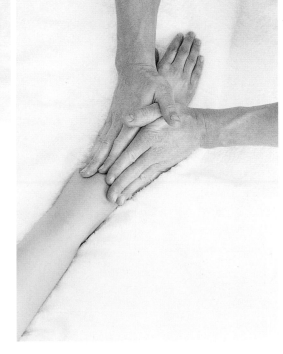

9 | To finish, place the arm on the floor and use both hands to effleurage up the whole arm. When you reach the shoulder, slide your outer hand beneath the arm, sandwiching the arm between your hands. Then glide your hands down the arm and pull away at the fingertips. Repeat several times on both arms.

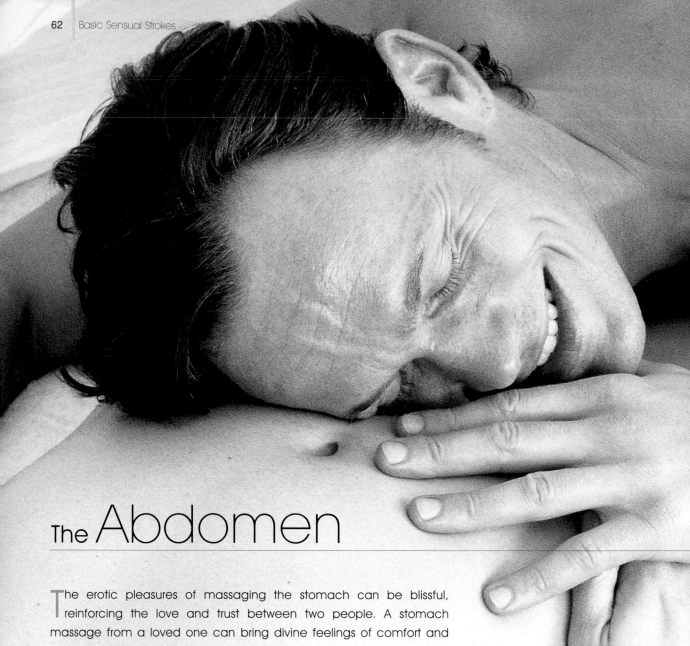

The Abdomen

The erotic pleasures of massaging the stomach can be blissful, reinforcing the love and trust between two people. A stomach massage from a loved one can bring divine feelings of comfort and peace, and a highly seductive sensation will flow through the whole body. Giving a stomach massage can be a wonderful experience as you allow your hands to explore and caress the beautiful, sensual curves and the soft, luscious skin, or strong, firm muscles. Tease the mysteriously sexual belly button to arouse and seduce, and to create feelings of connection between two people.

The abdomen is also a very sensitive and vulnerable area to work on, so caring, loving, warm hands are needed, especially at your first touch. Your partner will be very sensitive to this, and it will reflect on the rest of the massage.

Effleurage

Kneel beside your partner's abdomen, facing their head. Before you start your massage notice your partner's breathing and, as they breathe out, gently rest your hands either side of the abdomen. Hold this position for a few moments to allow your partner to become accustomed to your hands.

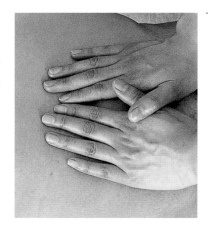

1 Glide your hands from the starting position so they rest on the stomach, fingers pointing toward your partner's head. Slowly slide your hands up over the lower rib cage. Separate your hands, and draw them down the sides.

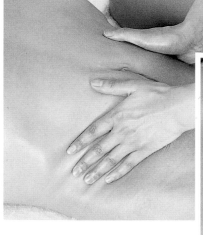

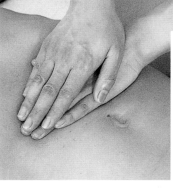

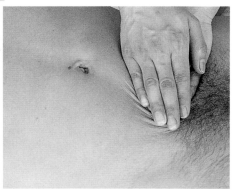

2 Turn the heels of your hands inward and bring them up to the starting position. Repeat this stroke to create an organic flowing movement over the abdomen.

3 Turn to face your partner's stomach. Place your hands gently on your partner's stomach, one on top of the other.

4 In a clockwise direction, slide your hands over and around the stomach, molding them over the far side before drawing them back to the starting position. The pressure should be firm but not too heavy.

Kneading

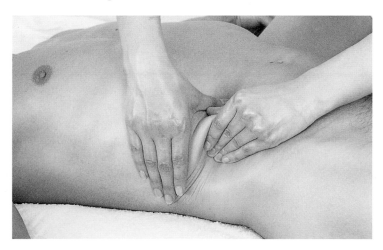

1 Lean over your partner and rest your open hands on the side of the stomach. Use one hand to glide along, and scoop up the flesh, squeezing and releasing before repeating with the opposite hand. Knead the stomach from the top to the bottom. Move your hands to the near side. Repeat the stroke, starting at the bottom of the stomach. Finish with effleurage.

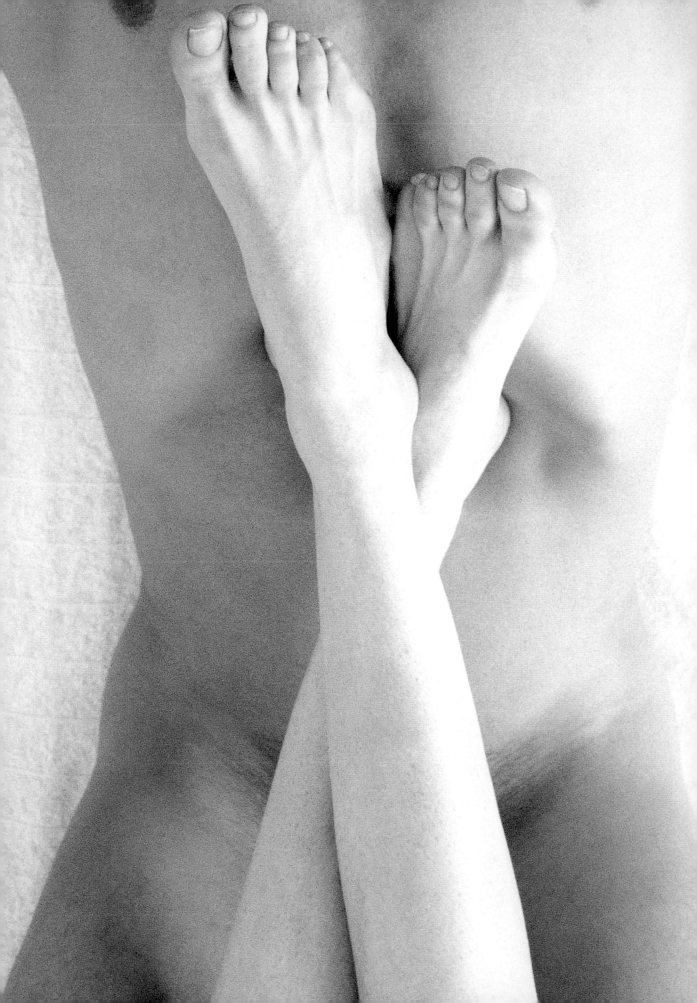

The Legs and Feet

Having aroused sensations all over your partner's body, allow that flow of feeling to continue downward by massaging the front of their legs and feet. Whether you have massaged the whole body, or just a section, squeezing, stroking, and caressing your partner's legs and feet is a wonderful way to finish a massage. Those strong powerful thighs with sensual, fleshy areas and the delicate ankle that flows into the soft curves of the foot all cry out to be stroked and squeezed. Linger in the luxury of seeing your partner lying in a state of bliss as you caress, play with, and lick their feet and toes, allowing the divine sensations to run through their whole body. Having your feet massaged can be deeply relaxing and sexual, and will calm the mind and body all at once.

Front of Leg Effleurage

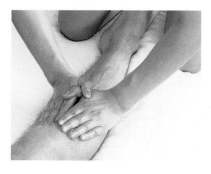

1   Kneel astride your partner's leg. Place your flat hands, index fingers together and pointing up the leg, on the ankle. Glide your hands up the leg. At the top of the thigh separate your hands to the sides and caress the muscles as you draw back down the leg.

2   Cup your hands around the lower part of your partner's leg, with your fingers in opposite directions. Move your hands back and forward, gradually working up the leg.

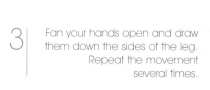

3   Fan your hands open and draw them down the sides of the leg. Repeat the movement several times.

Wringing

1   Kneel beside your partner's upper leg, and place both hands flat on the thigh, just above the knee. With the heels of your hands together, wrap your fingers around the leg. Slowly draw the heel of one hand toward your fingers and push the other hand away, creating a wringing movement. Slowly work up and down the whole of each thigh

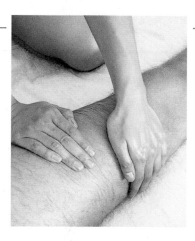

Kneading the Thigh

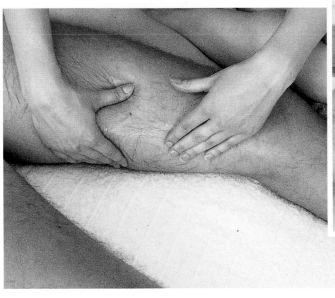

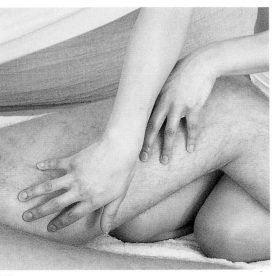

2 | Finish with effleurage strokes, this time bringing your hands right down to the feet and sandwiching the base and top of the foot between your hands before releasing at the toes.

1 | Sit to the side of your partner's leg and rest your flat, open hands on the inner thigh. Glide one hand along to scoop up the flesh between your thumb and index finger. Squeeze, release, and repeat with your other hand, kneading the whole inner thigh and top of the thigh from knee to groin.

Effleurage on the Feet

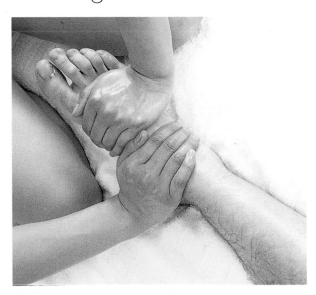

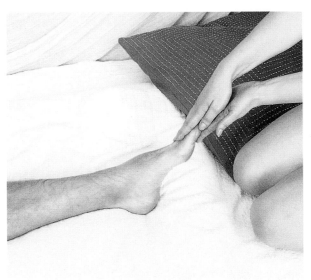

1 | Place your partner's foot between your knees and cup your hands over the foot. Slowly slide your hands over the foot to the lower leg. Fan your hands around the foot, one hand underneath and the other on top.

2 | Sandwich the foot between the palms of your hands. Squeeze the hands as you draw them up toward the toes. Tease and linger at the tip of the toes before pulling off. Repeat as one flowing movement.

Petrissage on the Feet

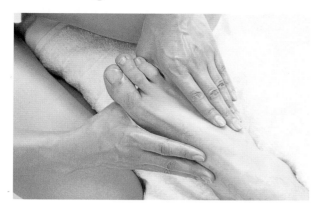

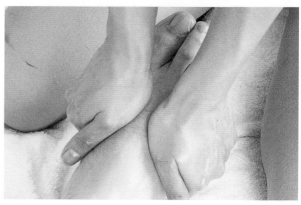

1 | With fingers facing the ankle either side of the foot, use firm pressure to slowly massage the top, sides, and ankle with circular motions. Keep your fingers together but do move your hands and thumbs to a comfortable position if you need.

2 | Wrap your hands around the foot, heels of the hands together. Slowly push the heels of your hands in an outward direction over the top of the foot. Lift your hands away and repeat the stroke.

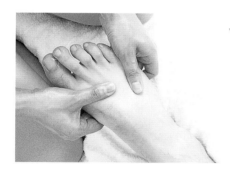

3 | Using your thumbs rotate the pads in small, firm circles over the top of the foot and ankle in one slow, movement.

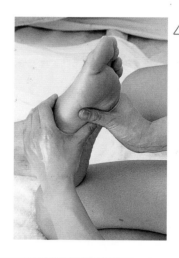

4 | Position yourself with your partner's foot on your knee and wrap your hands around the foot. Using your thumbs massage the underside of the foot in small circular motions, applying a firm pressure.

5 | Place one thumb above the other, just below the toes, and draw them out to each side of the foot. Release before repeating the stroke. Slowly move down the foot and back up to the starting position.

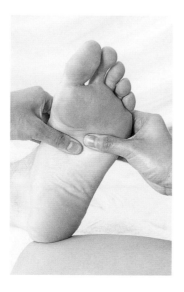

6 | Now, hold each toe and gently rotate in a circular motion. Repeat on each toe. Complete the massage using effleurage strokes up and down the leg and over the foot.

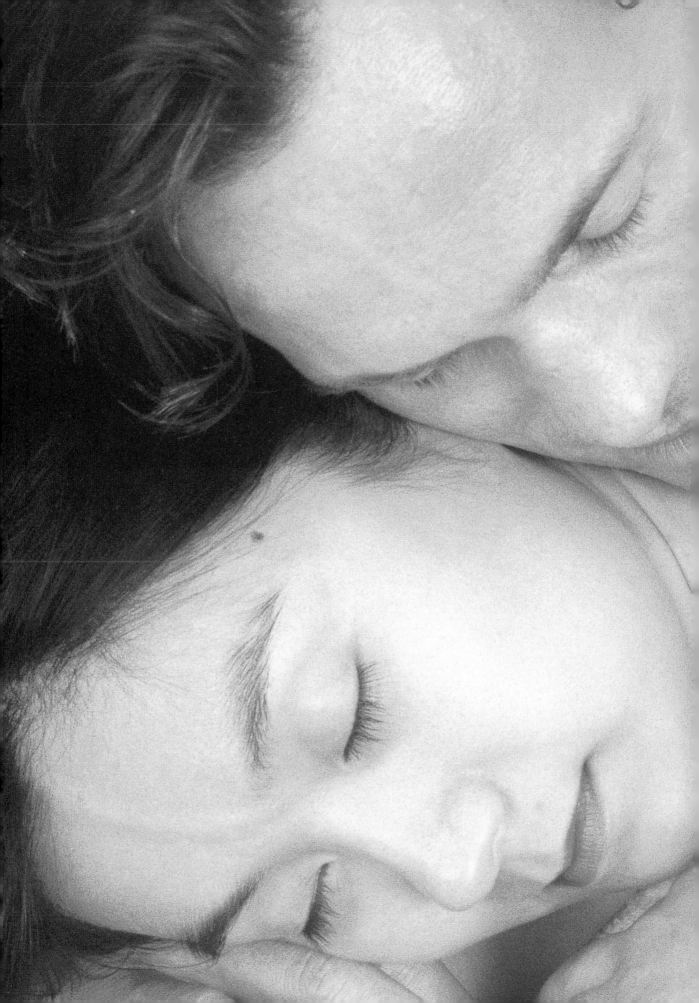

CHAPTER 3
Massaging your Partner

In an increasingly busy world massage is an excellent way of slowing down the pace of life and spending some intimate time with your partner.

It can reinforce the bonds of love and trust by communicating through touch, with a massage specifically created for the one you love. Using the techniques in Basic Sensual Strokes you can adapt a massage that you know your partner will appreciate. Choose one of the suggested recipes, specially designed for both men and women, using aromatherapy oils selected for their therapeutic properties. Experiment with jasmine, geranium, or palma rosa for a woman or choose the more woody fragrances of sandalwood, neroli, or vetiver for a man, Languish in their heady aromas while benefiting from their healing and rejuvenating effects. Formulated for hair, skin, and scalp, each recipe has a different characteristic which you can choose to suit your massage.

An important aspect of sensual massage is knowing the erogenous zones. Discover the sensitive areas of the skin such as the inside of the elbow, the toes, or the back of the neck. Paying particular attention to these areas can transport your partner into a dreamlike oasis. The beauty of massage is that you can apply it to everyday situations, adding zest and excitement to an otherwise ordinary routine. Using your partner's favorite oils and soaps you can transform a shave into an erotic experience they will never forget. For a woman there is nothing more relaxing than having her hair washed in the bath or a scalp massage to remove the stress of the day. The time spent together through massage, and the thought given to your partner, will make them feel adored and cherished, strengthening your relationship,

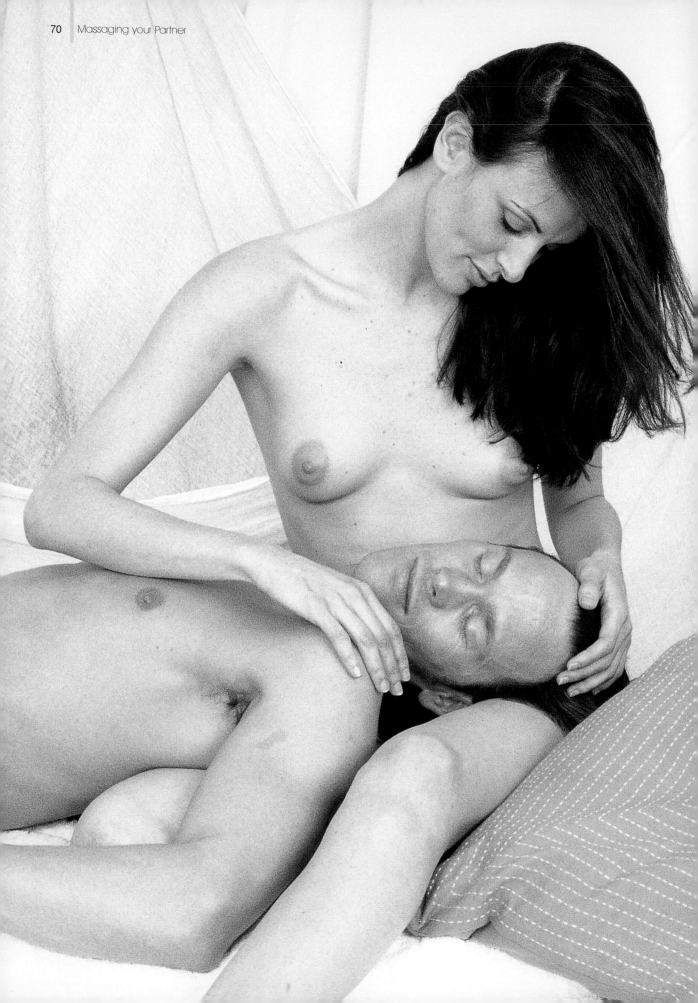

Massage for a Man

One of the most luxurious ways of giving your man a treat is to seduce him into the sensual pleasures of massage by washing him in a hot, steamy shower with luxurious soap and oils. Slowly massage and shave his face with rich shaving creams and oils, and pamper his body with warm oils. This will be a special time for both of you and a treat for him; a time when he can relax, unwind, and allow himself to do absolutely nothing except succumb to the sensual pleasures you are giving him.

The first thing to do is to prepare your room for massage by creating a calm environment away from your normal space. The ambience of the room is very important, as it should serve as a sanctuary, somewhere away from the pressures of everyday life. Begin by turning up the heat to keep your space cozy and warm. Keep the lighting low and soft, or simply burn candles. Choose "masculine" candles which are large and round. Scent the room by burning woody, earthy, and spicy oils such as sandalwood, vetiver, rosemary, clary sage or basil. Play gentle and soothing music, and cover the massage bed with blankets and cushions or with sumptuous fabrics in dark, rich colors.

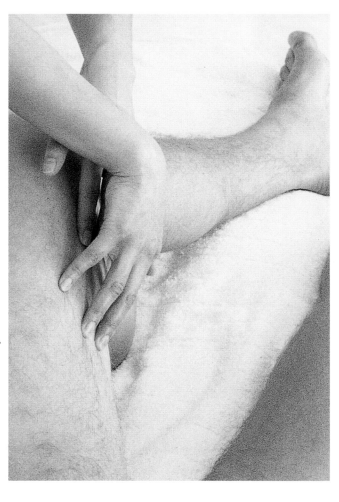

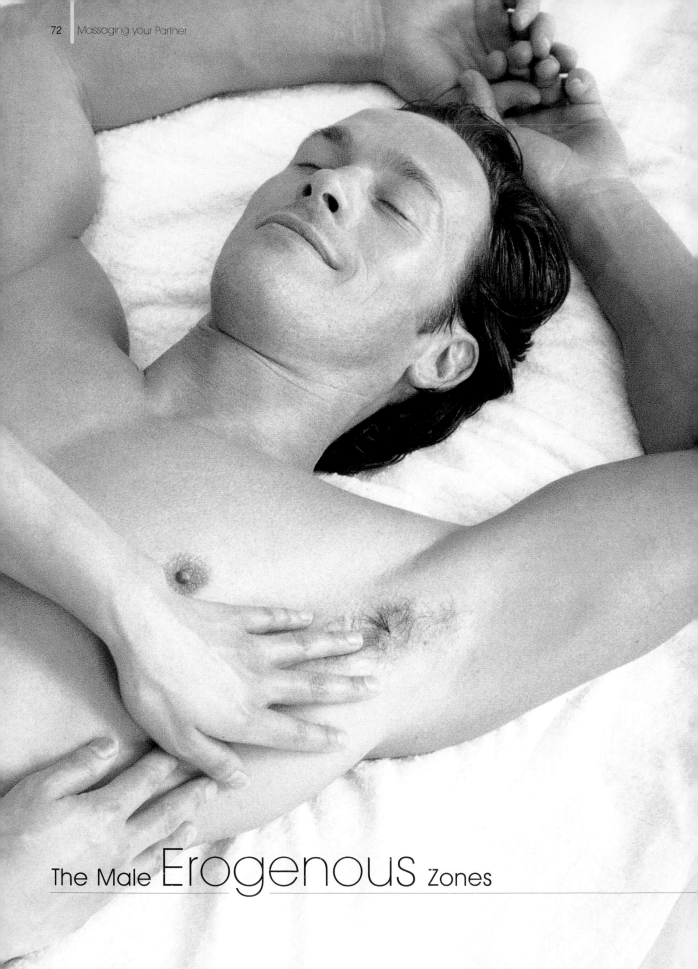

The Male Erogenous Zones

For a more erotic massage that will ignite the fires of passion, seductively kiss, lick or massage his erogenous zones to send shivers of delight through his whole body. Choose one of the sensual masculine recipes, or blend one of your own to massage him with. When you come to massage your partner, gently relax and soothe him with the basic sensual strokes. Tantalize and tease him by draping your hair over him, or using your nails to set his skin tingling. With sensual massage the whole body becomes an erogenous zone, however, specific areas are more sensitive for both men and women.

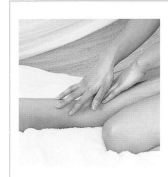

● THE INSIDE OF THE ELBOW

Gently stroke the inner part of the elbow for a dreamy, arousing effect. Continue toward the hand, finishing at the fingertips.

● THE DELICATE EARS AND LOBES

The ears are incredibly sensitive to touch, so be sure to caress them gently. Squeeze the lobes with your fingers, or kiss and lick around the ear.

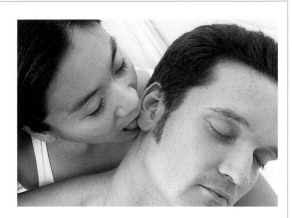

● THE KISSABLE NIPPLES

You can tantalize your man by sensually stroking an ice cube over his nipples, then licking, kissing, and sucking this most erotic of areas.

● THE POWERFUL, FLESHY INNER THIGH

Massaging the strong thighs, with their sensual areas, will make the hairs stand on end. Delight your partner by caressing the contours of the muscles, and kissing the soft flesh.

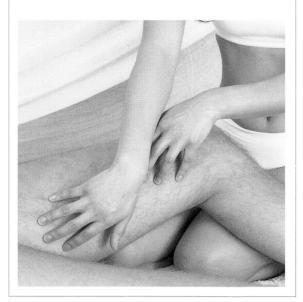

Aromatherapy Recipes for Men

These recipes have been created for you to use for any of the massage sequences but especially for men. They contain fresh, green, woody aromas, and when mixed with the suggested base oils are particularly luxurious. They are beneficial for the skin and general well-being. For the skin blend between 4—6 drops—depending on the skin's sensitivity—with two thirds of a tablespoon (10ml) of base oil for the face. Increase this ratio for a body massage. For the scalp massage use either the oil or, alternatively, use one tablespoon (15ml) of orange water. Cover the scalp and leave for 15 minutes, before washing out thoroughly with shampoo.

Dry Skin

BASE OIL:
jojoba, avocado, or wheat germ

AROMATHERAPY OIL:
frankincense, sandalwood, or neroli

Normal Skin

BASE OIL:
avocado or almond

AROMATHERAPY OIL:
sandalwood, lemon, or lavender

Oily Skin

BASE OIL:
almond, grapeseed, or hazelnut

AROMATHERAPY OIL:
cypress, lemon, or lavender

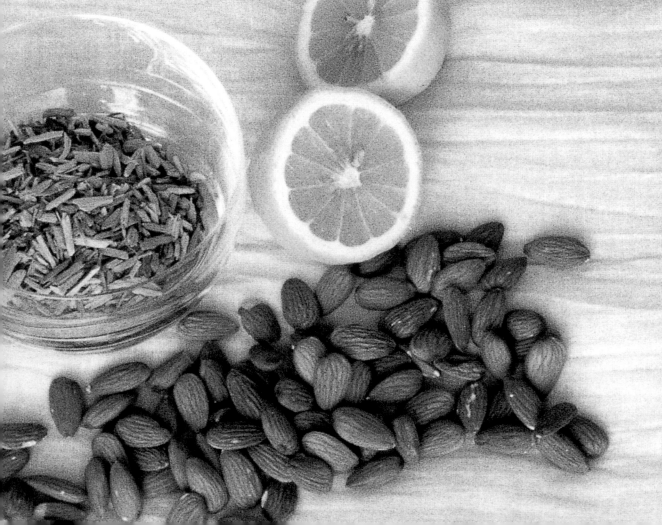

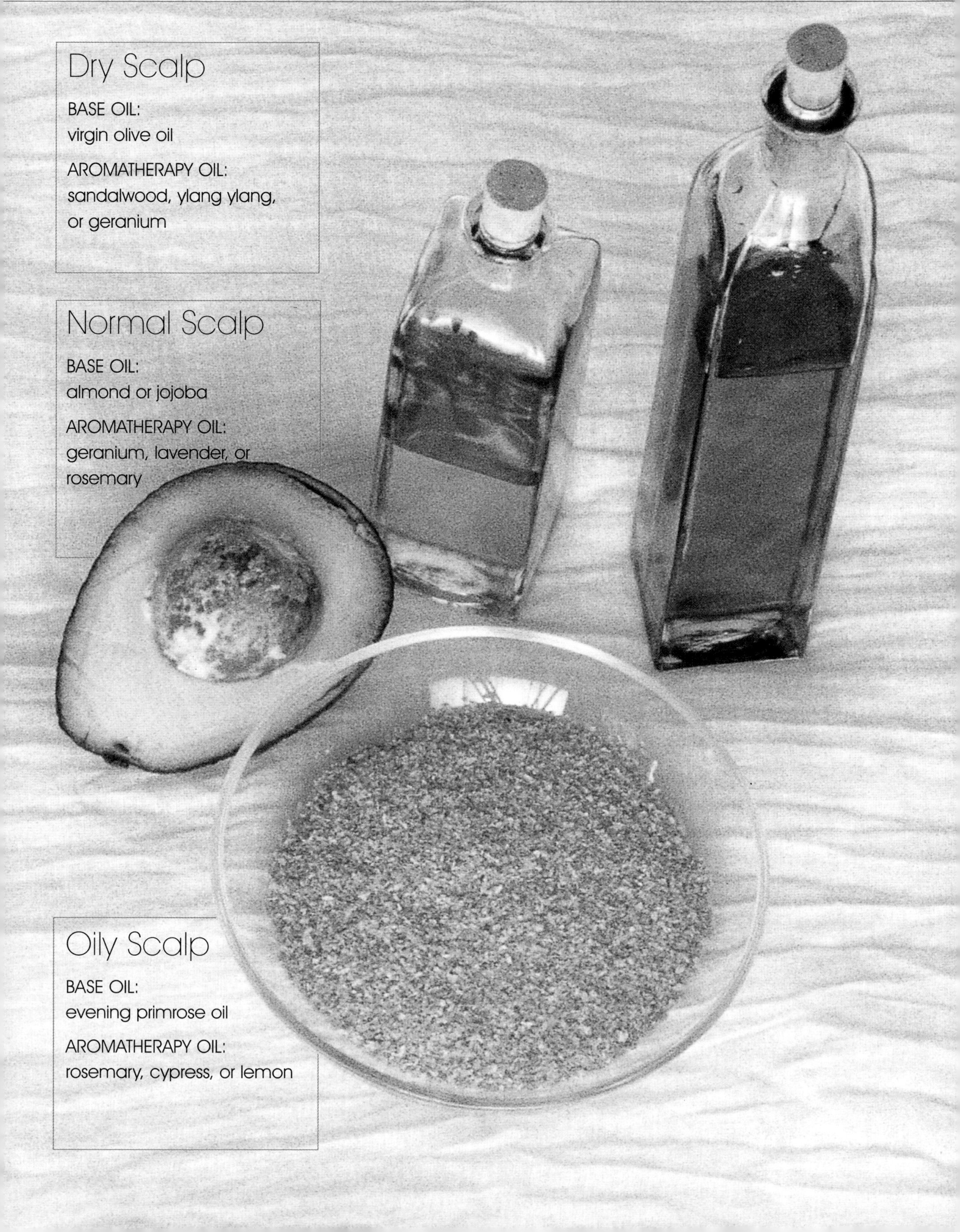

Dry Scalp

BASE OIL:
virgin olive oil

AROMATHERAPY OIL:
sandalwood, ylang ylang,
or geranium

Normal Scalp

BASE OIL:
almond or jojoba

AROMATHERAPY OIL:
geranium, lavender, or
rosemary

Oily Scalp

BASE OIL:
evening primrose oil

AROMATHERAPY OIL:
rosemary, cypress, or lemon

Shaving your
Partner

Before you start shaving your partner, gently lie him on his back on the floor in a comfortable position, and use the facial oils to lovingly and sensually massage his face using the basic sensual facial massage strokes.

If he has never received a facial massage before, allow a little time for him to relax and enjoy the sensation it will create.

If he has stubble, or a beard, still work upon this area but take a little bit longer to work the oils into the hair. Once he feels your soothing, sensual hands on his face he can relax and let the worries of the day drift away. Turn his usual shaving routine into something special and sensual. Buy a luxury shaving cream or gel with a delicious fragrance and natural ingredients or choose a seductive aftershave balm. Treat him to his favorite cologne, or use one that you will love to smell on him.

To shave him, sit him on the side of the bath or in a chair, keeping all the

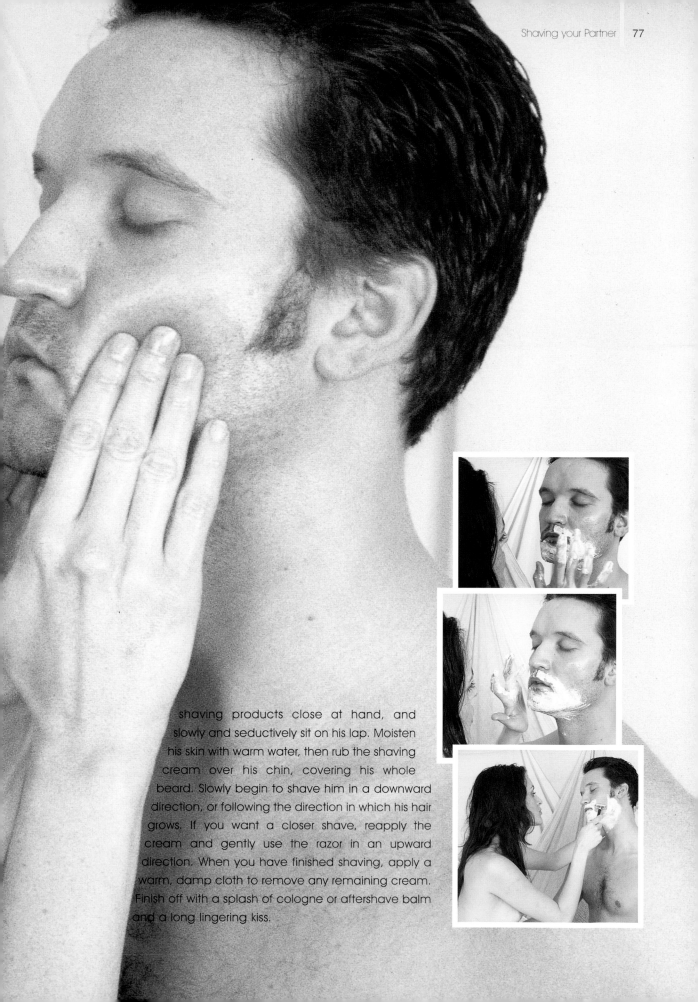

shaving products close at hand, and slowly and seductively sit on his lap. Moisten his skin with warm water, then rub the shaving cream over his chin, covering his whole beard. Slowly begin to shave him in a downward direction, or following the direction in which his hair grows. If you want a closer shave, reapply the cream and gently use the razor in an upward direction. When you have finished shaving, apply a warm, damp cloth to remove any remaining cream. Finish off with a splash of cologne or aftershave balm and a long lingering kiss.

Showering Together

Turn your bathroom into a sanctuary of pleasure that your man will love. Pre-warm the bathroom, soften its appearance with glowing candlelight, and scent the air with woody and spicy oils, such as bergamot, basil, or cedarwood. Add to the ambience and make the room sumptuous with cushions, pillows, and warm towels. Treat him to a glass of his favorite wine or champagne.

Before you shower him, make a luxurious sensual massage oil mixture with an intoxicating masculine fragrance. Give him a gift, such as an extra-special soap or shower gel especially for washing him with, and then slowly and seductively undress him and pre-warm the shower. Allow him to stand underneath for a few moments, enjoying the water as it falls over his body, relaxing his muscles.

Join him in the shower, holding him close to you, allowing a few moments of pleasure together as the warm water cascades off each of your bodies. Using the soap, make a lather in your hands and start to wash and caress his whole body. Use slow, circular movements then allow the water to rinse off the lather. When his skin is clean stand behind your partner and use the massage oil to gently but firmly squeeze and knead his shoulders, allowing the water to spread the oils down the body. Using the rest of the oil, start to massage his body using sensual squeezing or caressing strokes, strokes which feel pleasing to him. You can try using your whole body to rub against him as the sensation of two wet and oiled bodies moving together is highly erotic. When you have completed your massage, allow yourself a few moments together enjoying the heady fragrance from the oils, which the steam will diffuse, and then step out from the shower. Dry him from top to toe with soft, warm towels.

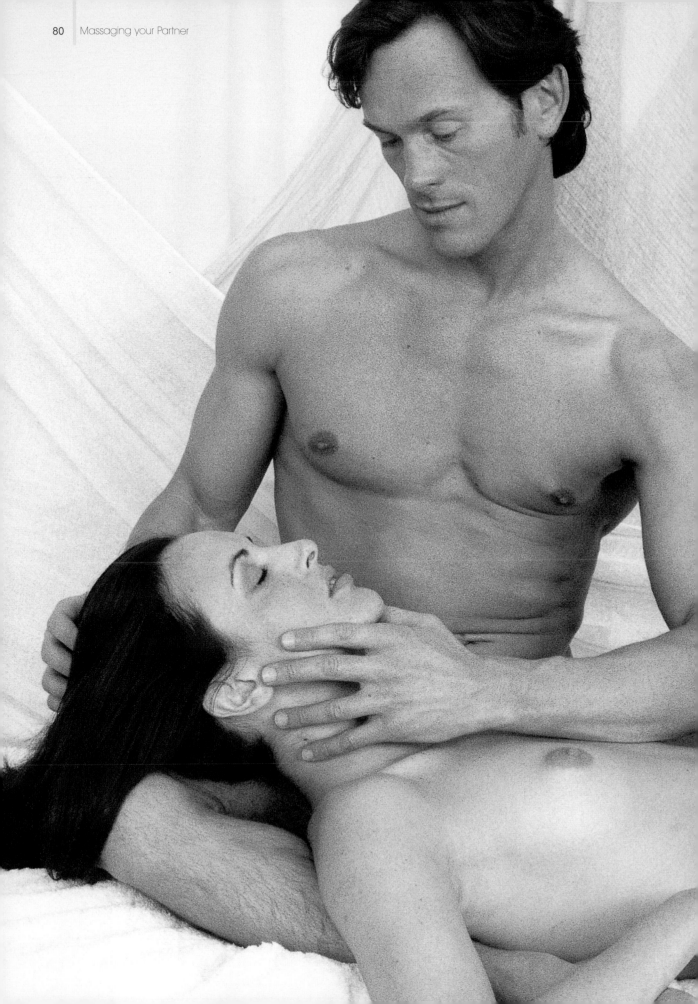

Massage for a Woman

Women love to be pampered and adored, and one of the most pleasurable treats you can give your partner is to bathe her in sensuous, fragrant oils and then to wash her hair with rich, luxurious shampoos and conditioners. You could massage her scalp using specially prepared oils. Or try teasing her skin with silks, flowers, and heady perfumed massage oils, taking nothing in return except the sheer enjoyment of pleasing her with the sensual feelings and experiences you are creating for her.

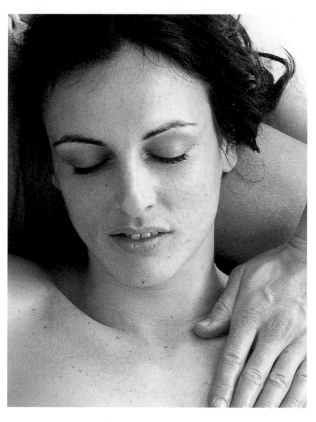

Before inviting her in, turn the room in which you're going to massage into a chamber of paradise fit for a goddess.

Use soft, gentle colors to decorate the chamber, and fill the room with a flickering warm glow from burning candles. Intoxicate the air with heady fragrances such as ylang ylang, jasmine, or mimosa. Make the massage feel sumptuous and sensual with cool, white sheets or soft blankets. Decorate the room with her favorite flowers, which will also fill the air with their subtle aroma. Tempt her with delicious tropical fruits placed around the room, and play soft, sensual music for her. When this setting has been created ask her to lie on the massage bed, make sure she is comfortable, and then begin your massage.

The Female Erogenous Zones

With its sinuous curves and delicate skin the female body has a plethora of erogenous zones. By stroking and licking different areas you can discover the parts that arouse your partner the most. Take time between massage strokes to caress sensitive areas of the body that you know she will love, to heighten the overall effect of the massage. Choose from the soft, tender nipples, the ticklish toes, and the nape of the neck. Experiment to find your partner's preferences and learn more about her body.

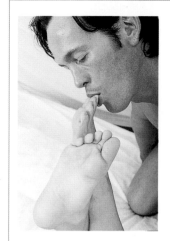

TICKLISH TOES

The feet, and especially the toes, are extremely sensitive. Use a feather or piece of fabric to draw between the toes and across the feet. Kiss them and blow on the skin to create an extra sensation.

THE TENDER NIPPLES

The most obvious of erogenous zones, the nipple is highly sensitive. Brushing the delicate nipple and surrounding area can send shivers of delight through your partner's body.

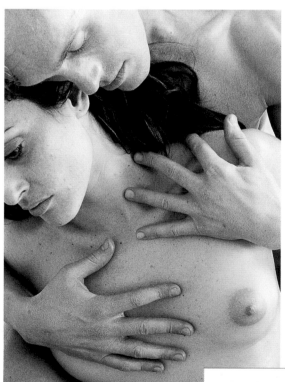

THE NAPE OF THE NECK

The nape of the neck conceals a soft down-like hair that will stand on end if caressed. An excellent place to stroke to express love and intimacy.

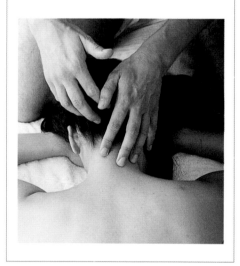

THE SENSITIVE CURVE OF THE BACK

When lightly stroked this erogenous zone sends a wave of pleasure up the spine. Brush across the buttocks for an added thrill.

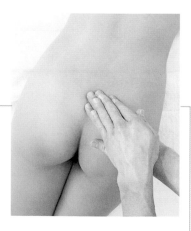

Aromatherapy Recipes for Women

These recipes have been specially created with women in mind, using heady floral fragrances. Use when washing the hair or try the skin recipes for a face or body massage. Blend 4—6 drops of a single oil, or combination of oils to two thirds of a tablespoon (10ml) of base oil for a face massage.

Increase the ratio for a body massage. For the hair use one tablespoon (15ml) as a base, then add the specified aromatherapy oils, leave for 15 minutes and then rinse thoroughly. Alternatively, use orange water instead of oil for the hair.

Normal Hair

BASE OIL:
almond

AROMATHERAPY OIL:
- 6 drops lavender
- 6 drops geranium

Oily Hair

BASE OIL:
peach kernal

AROMATHERAPY OIL:
- 6 drops lavender
- 6 drops cypress
- 6 drops lemon

Dry Hair

BASE OIL:
jojoba or virgin olive oil

AROMATHERAPY OIL:
- 6 drops lavender
- 8 drops sandalwood
- 6 drops rosemary

Final Rinse

Use 2—3 drops of one of the following per pint (½ l) of water:

NORMAL HAIR:
lavender, geranium, orange, lemon, or rosemary

DRY HAIR:
lavender, ylang ylang, sandalwood, or rose

OILY HAIR:
lemon, lavender, rosemary, or frankincense

Normal Skin

BASE OIL:
jojoba, almond, or evening primrose

AROMATHERAPY OIL:
lavender, rose, or geranium

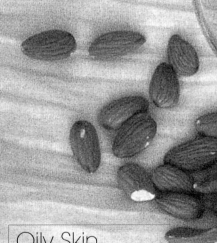

Oily Skin

BASE OIL:
grapeseed, hazelnut, or almond

AROMATHERAPY OIL:
lavender, geranium, or palma rosa

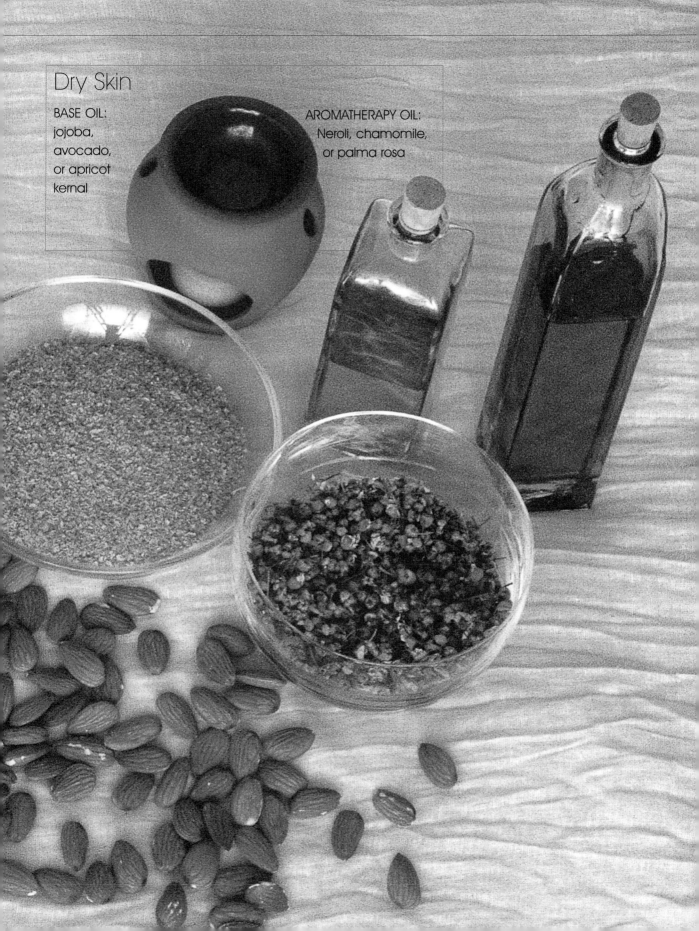

Dry Skin

BASE OIL:
jojoba,
avocado,
or apricot
kernal

AROMATHERAPY OIL:
Neroli, chamomile,
or palma rosa

Washing her Hair

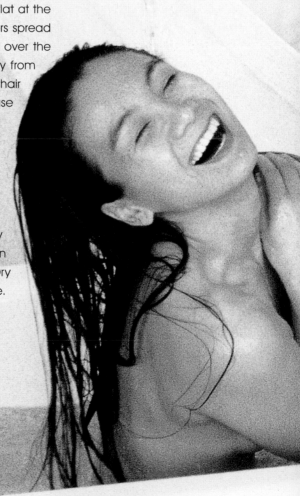

One of the most pleasurable and sensual experiences for a woman is to have her hair washed using her favorite shampoo, or a blend of aromatic essentail oils. What can otherwise be a routine chore becomes a great pleasure when she can relax and let you do the work. Before washing her hair, create a mixture of aromatic oils to massage into her hair and scalp, which will give her hair luster and shine, and an intoxicating smell. You can wash your partner's hair with her either sitting in the bath, or sitting alongside the bath with her head tilted gently back.

Wet the hair, then apply the shampoo or oil working it in gently. Starting at the hairline, massage the scalp with your fingertips, using small circular movements. Slowly work your way along the scalp to the back of the head, before returning to the front hairline. Continue this motion then repeat, starting at the side of the face. Now place one hand flat at the base of her neck, and the other at the forehead with the fingers spread open and pointing towards the other hand. Draw your hands over the scalp until your fingers interlock, then lift the hair upwards away from the head. Using your fingertips or nails, comb your partner's hair from root to tip. Start at the front hairline and run down to the base of the neck, following one hand smoothly after the other.

Massage the whole scalp with large circular movements using the flat pads of your outspread fingers. If you have used a hair oil, it is a good idea to wrap her hair in a warm towel and leave it on for about 10 minutes. Then shampoo and rinse. To finish, add a few drops of aromatherapy oil to cool water, rinse and then wrap her hair in a warm towel. Dry her hair to complete the massage.

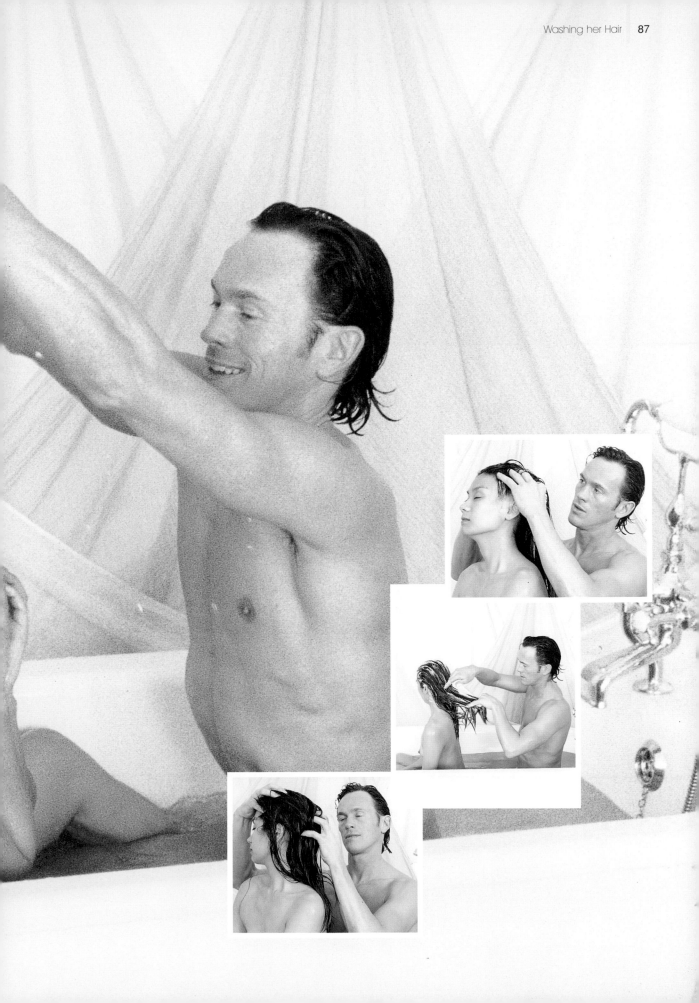

Scalp Massage

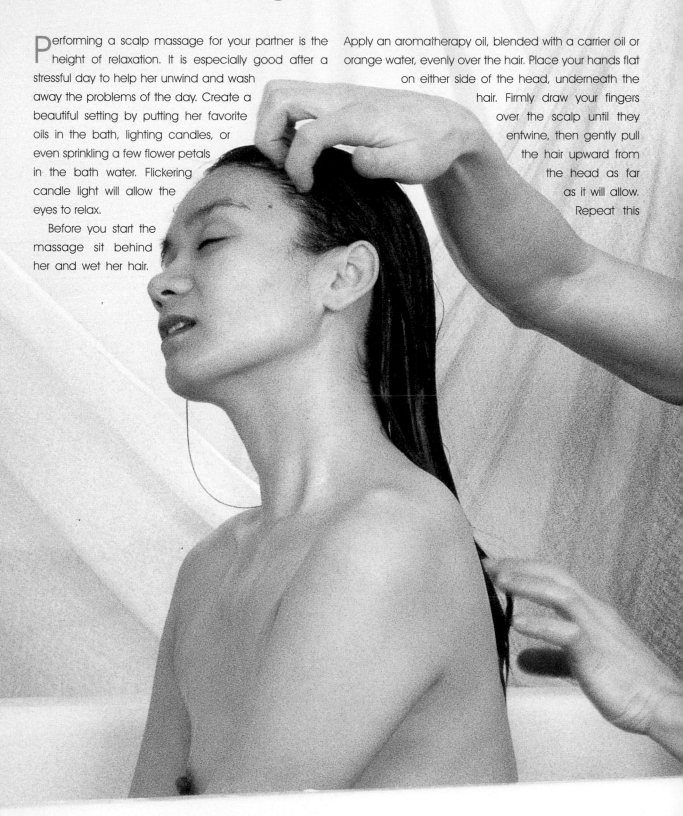

Performing a scalp massage for your partner is the height of relaxation. It is especially good after a stressful day to help her unwind and wash away the problems of the day. Create a beautiful setting by putting her favorite oils in the bath, lighting candles, or even sprinkling a few flower petals in the bath water. Flickering candle light will allow the eyes to relax.

Before you start the massage sit behind her and wet her hair.

Apply an aromatherapy oil, blended with a carrier oil or orange water, evenly over the hair. Place your hands flat on either side of the head, underneath the hair. Firmly draw your fingers over the scalp until they entwine, then gently pull the hair upward from the head as far as it will allow. Repeat this action several times. Now repeat this stroke working from the base of the neck up toward the forehead. Now repeat this stroke from the base of the neck upward, and from the forehead working backward. Place the pads of your

fingers on the front and back hairline and massage the scalp using small circular motions. Work from the hairline across the top of the scalp. Repeat this motion on both sides of the head above the ears. To finish the massage draw your fingernails from the hairline back down the head toward the base of the neck running your fingers through her hair. Repeat this stroke several times for the ultimate relaxation.

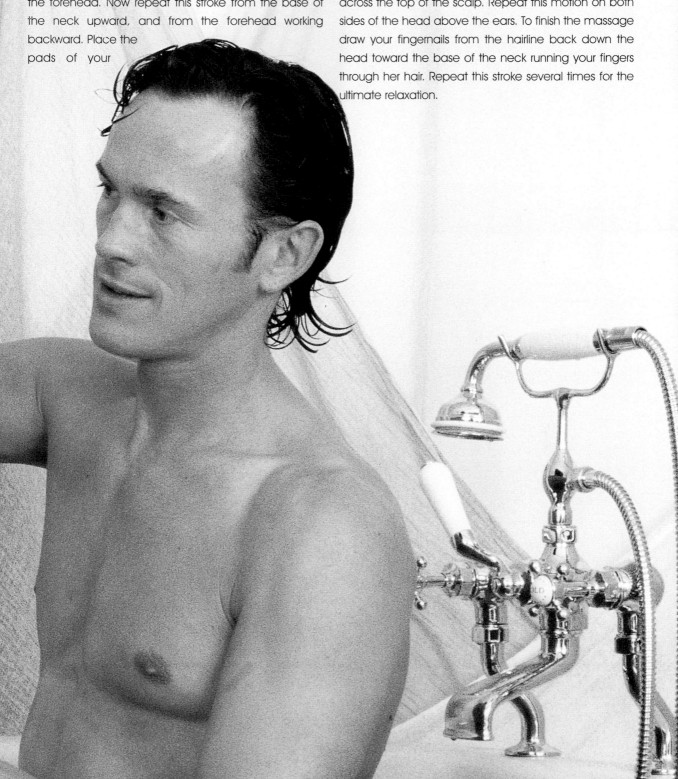

CHAPTER 4
Massage from Around the World

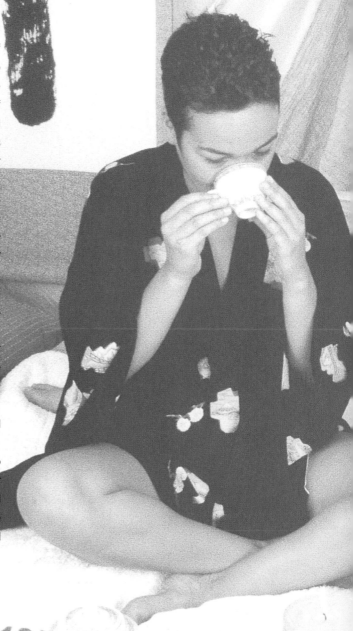

Since ancient items, many cultures have used massage for the promotion of health, for the art of seduction, and for the pure pleasure of bringing two people together. To complement the massage, there would be rituals and dances, and the preparation of exquisite oils. The Native Indians of America played powerful music to enhance the massage, using drums to create a hypnotic rhythm that would flow through their bodies, allowing the sensual spirit to awaken.

Setting the scene for your massage can be a magical experience. Choose a favorite part of the world, and recreate your memories by turning the massage room into a place of fantasy. Your sensual play will be heightened by the atmosphere of a far off land, such as India with its luxurious fabrics, rich colors, and mystical fragrances. Treat your partner to delicious foods and drinks from their favorite country.

The different massages will allow you and your partner to experiment. You may choose the sensual massage from Egypt, with its long, flowing strokes and luxurious oils, or you may prefer the tranquil massage of the chakras, used in India to open up powerful energy centers, and allow sensual energy to flow through the body.

All the massage techniques have been chosen to complement each other. You may take one particular technique and incorporate it into your basic sensual massage. Whatever you choose, enjoy the experience of giving and receiving a sensual massage from around the world.

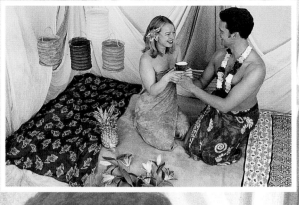

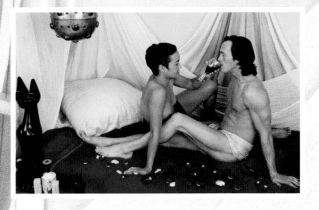

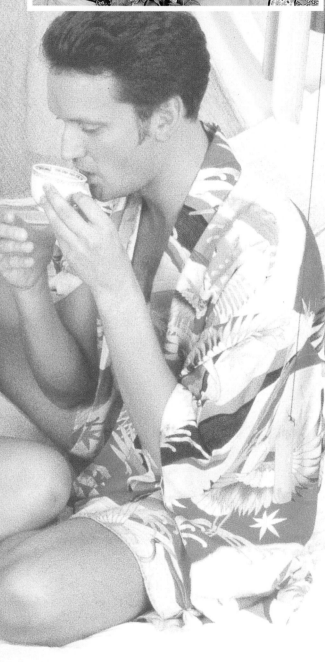

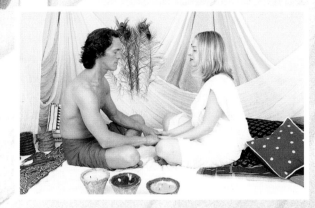

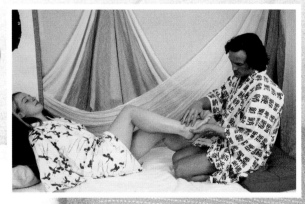

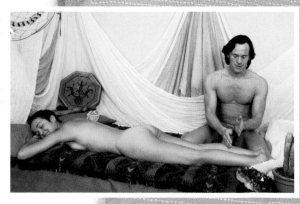

Left: massage set in China. Clockwise from top left:
massages set in Hawaii, Egypt, India, Japan, and
Native America.

Meditation and Massage from India

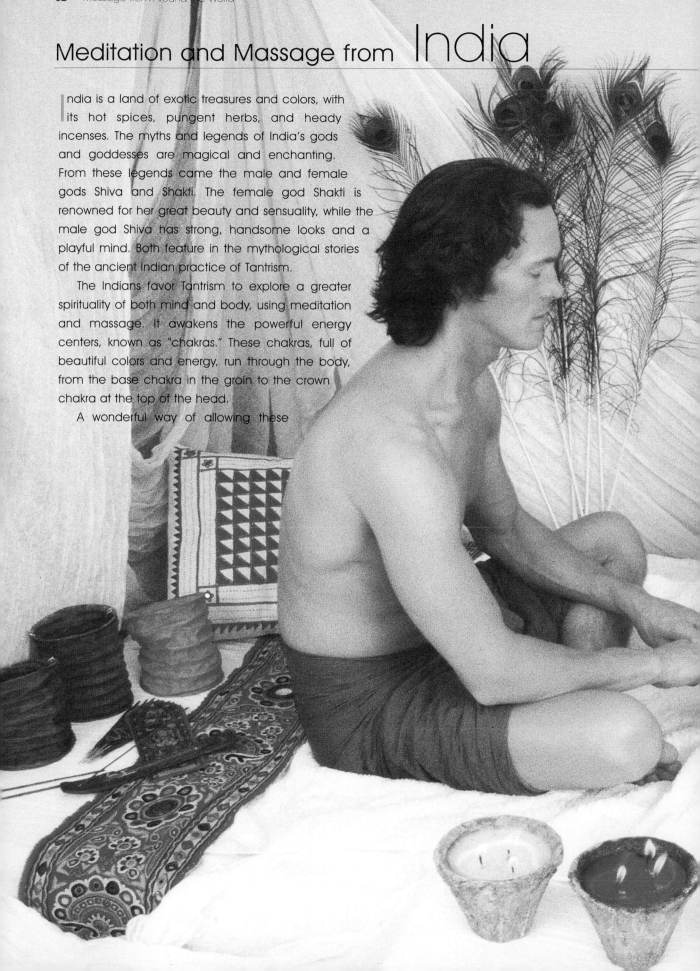

India is a land of exotic treasures and colors, with its hot spices, pungent herbs, and heady incenses. The myths and legends of India's gods and goddesses are magical and enchanting. From these legends came the male and female gods Shiva and Shakti. The female god Shakti is renowned for her great beauty and sensuality, while the male god Shiva has strong, handsome looks and a playful mind. Both feature in the mythological stories of the ancient Indian practice of Tantrism.

The Indians favor Tantrism to explore a greater spirituality of both mind and body, using meditation and massage. It awakens the powerful energy centers, known as "chakras." These chakras, full of beautiful colors and energy, run through the body, from the base chakra in the groin to the crown chakra at the top of the head.

A wonderful way of allowing these

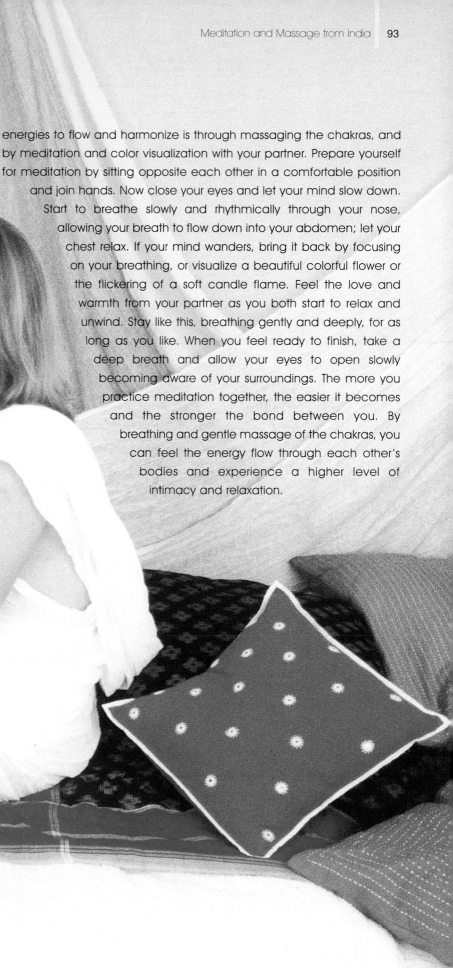

energies to flow and harmonize is through massaging the chakras, and by meditation and color visualization with your partner. Prepare yourself for meditation by sitting opposite each other in a comfortable position and join hands. Now close your eyes and let your mind slow down. Start to breathe slowly and rhythmically through your nose, allowing your breath to flow down into your abdomen; let your chest relax. If your mind wanders, bring it back by focusing on your breathing, or visualize a beautiful colorful flower or the flickering of a soft candle flame. Feel the love and warmth from your partner as you both start to relax and unwind. Stay like this, breathing gently and deeply, for as long as you like. When you feel ready to finish, take a deep breath and allow your eyes to open slowly becoming aware of your surroundings. The more you practice meditation together, the easier it becomes and the stronger the bond between you. By breathing and gentle massage of the chakras, you can feel the energy flow through each other's bodies and experience a higher level of intimacy and relaxation.

The Chakra Massage

The principle of chakra massage is to use meditation to concentrate positive energy to seven chakra centers. Refer to the picture opposite for their position and how they relate to the rest of the body.

1 Start by meditating sitting opposite each other. Concentrate your thoughts, allowing energy to flow between you. Lie your partner on their back and place your hands over the area of the base chakra, close your eyes and relax. Visualize a passionate red color flowing down your arms into your partner's chakra.

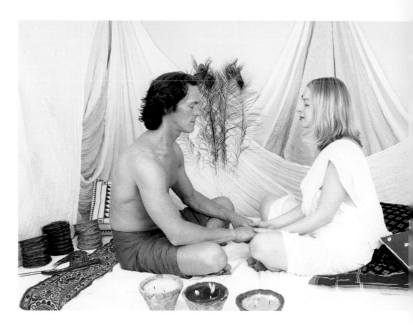

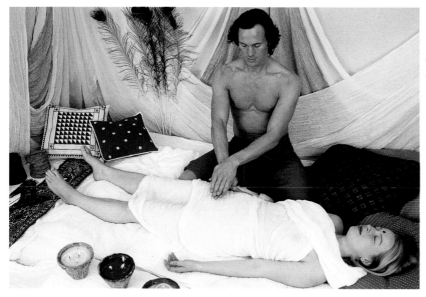

2 Stay like this for a few seconds before visualizing a beautiful red flower with closed petals. See the exquisite petals slowly opening to produce a flower. When you have finished the visualization, send thoughts of love and well-being to your partner. Take a few moments to relax before moving to the next chakra and its matching color.

3 As you work on each chakra, encourage your partner to visualize colors and images, using nature as inspiration. Finish at the crown chakra and remain for a few minutes. When both of your energies have been released try a gentle massage.

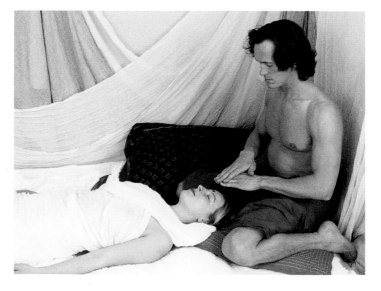

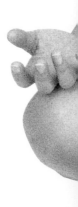

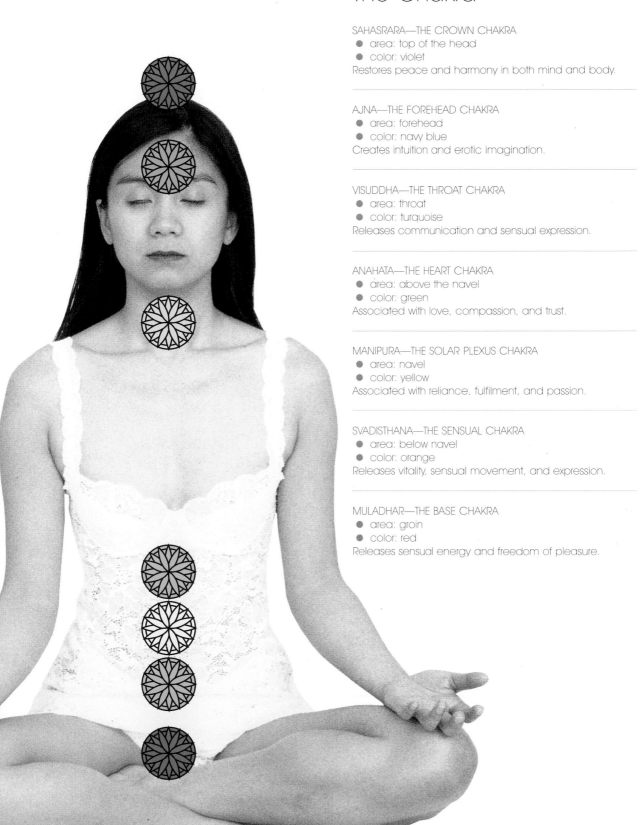

The Chakra

SAHASRARA—THE CROWN CHAKRA
- area: top of the head
- color: violet

Restores peace and harmony in both mind and body.

AJNA—THE FOREHEAD CHAKRA
- area: forehead
- color: navy blue

Creates intuition and erotic imagination.

VISUDDHA—THE THROAT CHAKRA
- area: throat
- color: turquoise

Releases communication and sensual expression.

ANAHATA—THE HEART CHAKRA
- area: above the navel
- color: green

Associated with love, compassion, and trust.

MANIPURA—THE SOLAR PLEXUS CHAKRA
- area: navel
- color: yellow

Associated with reliance, fulfilment, and passion.

SVADISTHANA—THE SENSUAL CHAKRA
- area: below navel
- color: orange

Releases vitality, sensual movement, and expression.

MULADHAR—THE BASE CHAKRA
- area: groin
- color: red

Releases sensual energy and freedom of pleasure.

Exotic Massage from Hawaii

Hawaii, the beautiful island of the orchids, with its soft, sandy beaches and warm, azure waters, is a paradise full of exotic sensual fruits, flowers, and gently waving palm trees. It is home to the ancient, spiritual, and powerful Kahuna priests who combined massage and meditation as a way of calming their minds and bodies. The well-being and long life of the Kahuna priests was greatly envied, and has been associated with their daily massage routine. This massage is still practiced in Hawaii and around the world, giving that same sense of good health, happiness, and tranquillity.

To recreate the setting of a Hawaiian tropical beach, fragrance the air with exotic oils such as vanilla, coconut,

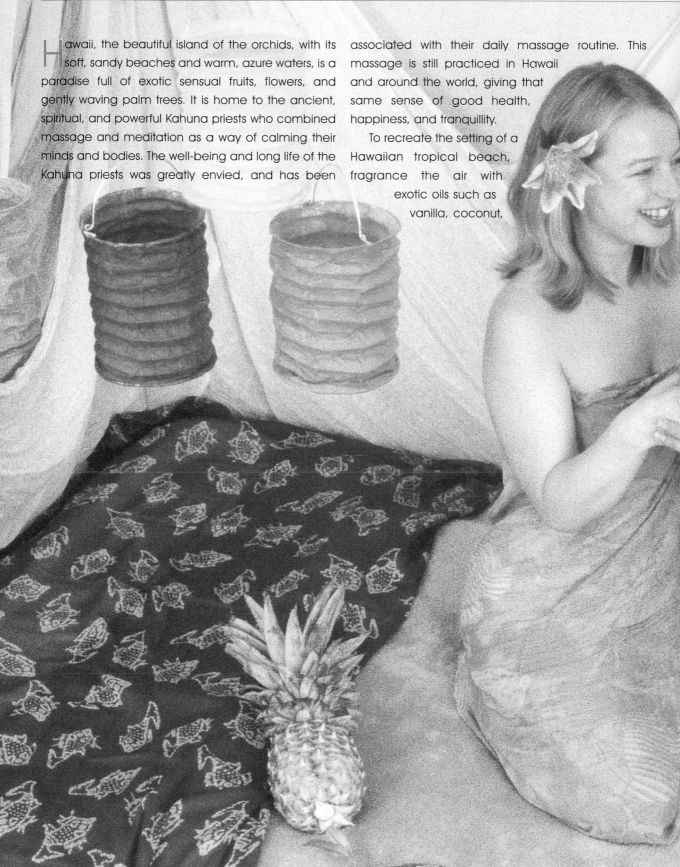

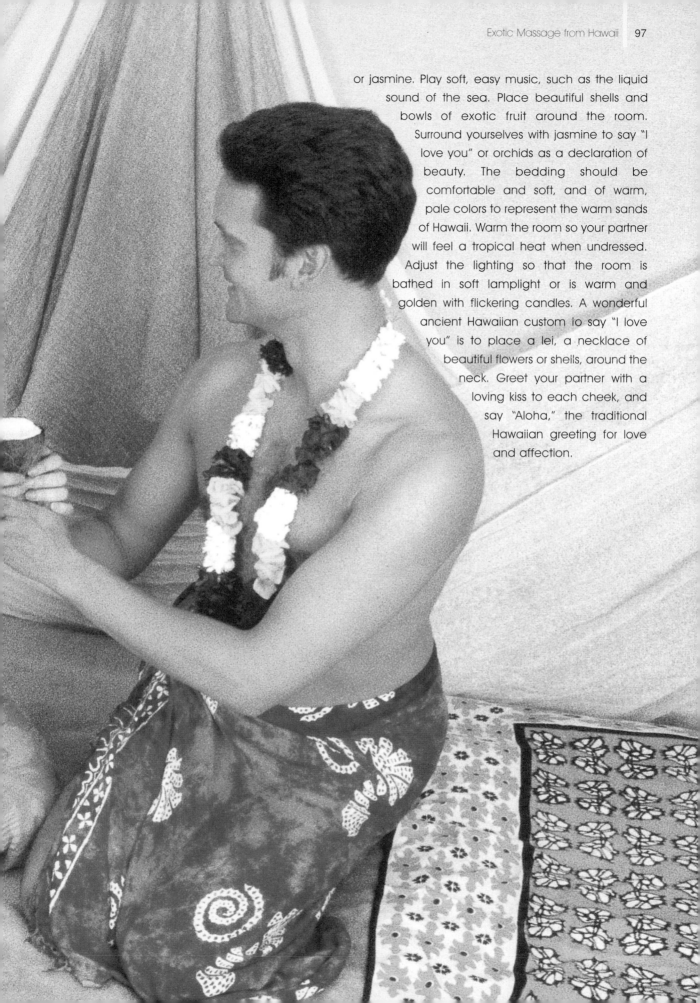

or jasmine. Play soft, easy music, such as the liquid sound of the sea. Place beautiful shells and bowls of exotic fruit around the room. Surround yourselves with jasmine to say "I love you" or orchids as a declaration of beauty. The bedding should be comfortable and soft, and of warm, pale colors to represent the warm sands of Hawaii. Warm the room so your partner will feel a tropical heat when undressed. Adjust the lighting so that the room is bathed in soft lamplight or is warm and golden with flickering candles. A wonderful ancient Hawaiian custom to say "I love you" is to place a lei, a necklace of beautiful flowers or shells, around the neck. Greet your partner with a loving kiss to each cheek, and say "Aloha," the traditional Hawaiian greeting for love and affection.

Arm Massage

Leading up to the massage offer a traditional Hawaiian cocktail made from exotic fruits and decorated with flowers, such as a Mai Tai with rum, orange curaçao, and lemon juice or a Blue Lagoon with vodka, blue curaçao, and lemon juice. Alternatively, mix a selection of tropical fruit juices for a non-alcoholic drink.

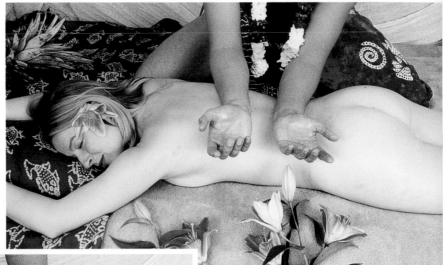

1 | Lie your partner on their stomach, arms out by their sides while you face the back. Rest the middle of your forearms, keeping your forearms flat on the skin. Slowly massage the back and buttocks by sweeping your arm in a circlular motion. Repeat with the other arm, then with both.

2 | Rest your forearms on the center of the back, and gently lean over. Move them in opposite directions with one arm gliding to the neck, and the other to the buttocks, ending at the top of the leg.

3 | Move alongside the body facing the upper thighs. Gently repeat the forearm movement, stroking across the top of the thighs up to the buttocks.

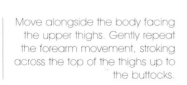

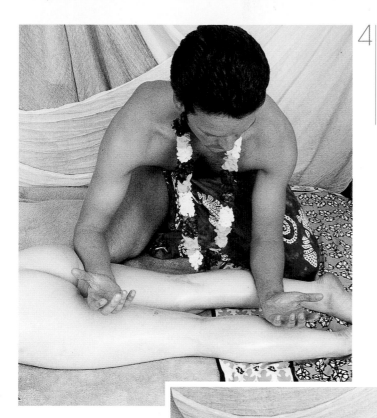

4 Now gently rest your forearms on either side the knees, and move both arms in different directions. Glide the first arm over the back of the thighs, and the other over the calves, gently stroking the back of the heels and brushing the arch of the foot.

5 Move up and kneel astride your partner's head. Rest your forearms on your partner's back on either side of the spine with palms facing upward. With small, circular motions, work your way down the back, being careful to maintain your balance. Complete the stroke by returning up the back.

6 Using the same technique continue with this stroke, but using alternate arms. Work up and down the back from the shoulders to the buttocks and back up again, taking care not to cause any strain.

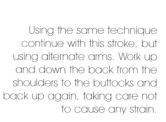

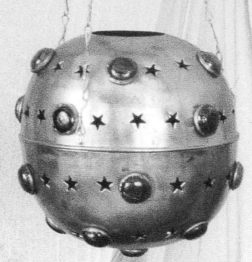

Soothing Massage from Egypt

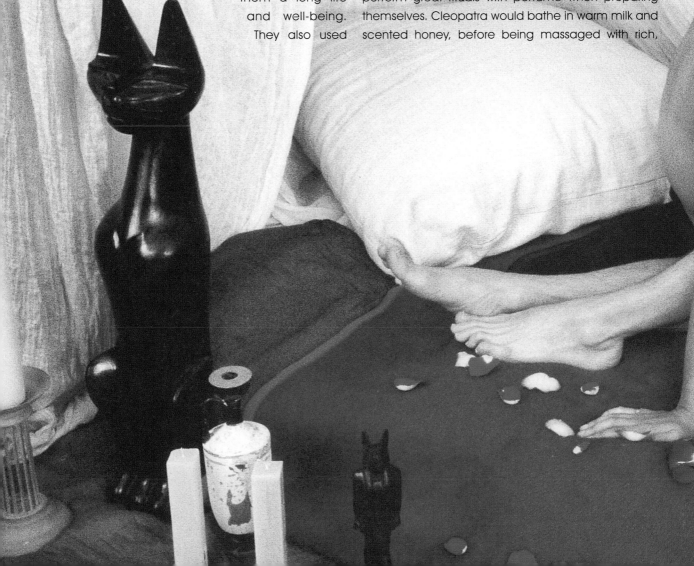

The ancient Egyptians were renowned for their love of bathing and massage. They used luscious oils made from flowers and herbs, which they believed would give them a long life and well-being. They also used their aphrodisiac qualities in the rituals of seduction.

The Egyptians placed great emphasis on the art of seduction and preparation, to enchant during love-making and to help entice a partner. They would perform great rituals with perfume when preparing themselves. Cleopatra would bathe in warm milk and scented honey, before being massaged with rich, luxurious oils full of aphrodisiac herbs and flowers. Her final preparations involved blending an intoxicatingly alluring mixture of oils, herbs, and flowers, which she would use to massage and arouse her partner.

The ancient Egyptians were also great believers in the powerful aphrodisiac properties of flowers and herbs for newly-wed couples. Beautiful, expensive flowers would be strewn on the wedding bed and around the room to impart their heady perfume and to intoxicate the newly weds. This allowed them to relax and release any inhibitions, and allow their sexuality to flow on their first night together.

To increase feelings of passion in your relationship, create an Egyptian chamber of desire. Make the room luxurious and rich by using sensual fabrics such as silks or satins to cover your massage surface. Light the room with beautiful glass oil burners, or place nightlights in specially made colored glass vases. To reinforce the mystical ambience of Egypt, perfume the air with oils and incense, such as frankincense, cedarwood, cinnamon, or rose, and scatter the petals of your partner's favorite flowers over the massage surface and around the room.

Lover's Massage

As your partner enters the chamber lead them to the massage bed and give them a glass of ruby red wine. When your partner has drunk the wine, lie them comfortably on their stomach and, with the oils near by, begin the massage.

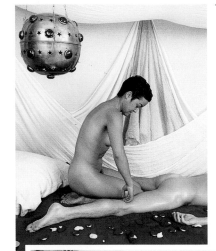

1 | Kneel between your partner's legs level with their knees. With both hands reaching backward, place the backs of your hands on their feet. Draw them up over the leg, rolling your hands over at the thighs. Glide up the legs, over the buttocks to the back. With a hand on each shoulder, stroke down the arms, then slide off at the fingers in one long stroke.

2 | Continue with this stroke, only this time using your fingernails to lightly scratch the surface of your partner's skin. Starting from your partner's hands, draw your nails up the arm, over the shoulders, and down the back, ending over the buttocks. Slide your hands as far down the back of the legs as you can reach.

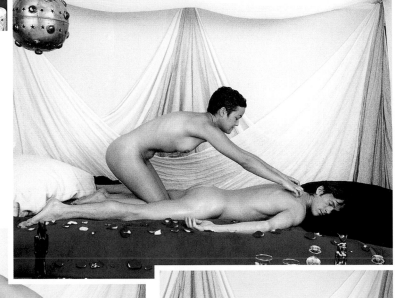

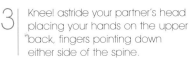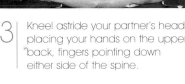

3 | Kneel astride your partner's head placing your hands on the upper back, fingers pointing down either side of the spine.

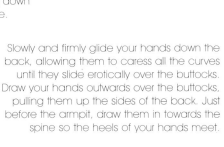

4 | Slowly and firmly glide your hands down the back, allowing them to caress all the curves until they slide erotically over the buttocks. Draw your hands outwards over the buttocks, pulling them up the sides of the back. Just before the armpit, draw them in towards the spine so the heels of your hands meet.

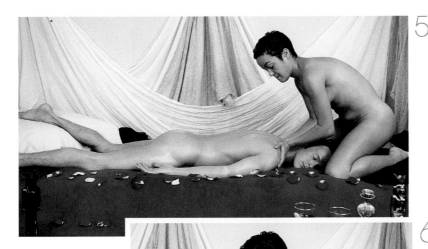

5 | Push your hands over the shoulders to the top of the arms, and glide them slowly down onto the hands. Linger on the palms. Then, stroking back up the arm over the shoulder, bring your hands underneath the shoulders, gliding them inwards and up the back of the neck and head.

6 | With your partner lying on their back, kneel astride their head. Place your palms, fingers pointing towards their feet, on your partner's breastbone. Glide your hands gently over the breast, brushing the nipples as you move over the stomach to the pubic bone. Fan your hands out over the hips, pulling them up the sides of the body through the armpits.

7 | Slide them over the chest, back to the starting position. From here, draw them out in a V-shape, with the heels of your hands leading across the upper chest, to the shoulder. Wrap your hands around the shoulders so your hands are underneath them, using your fingers to apply pressure.

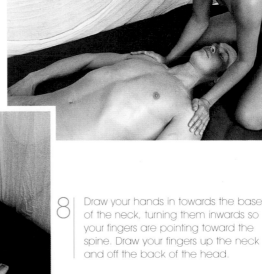

8 | Draw your hands in towards the base of the neck, turning them inwards so your fingers are pointing toward the spine. Draw your fingers up the neck and off the back of the head.

Foot Massage from Japan

The wonderfully sensual art of bathing your partner's feet, and massaging them with luxurious oils, can be one of the most arousing and soothing pleasures you can bestow. Foot massage has been performed through the ages by some of the most beautiful and serene geisha girls in Japan. Massaging the feet, using warm, scented water and gently perfumed soaps in beautiful, decorative bowls, was part of the ritual. When the feet had been washed, they would be dried in a soft, warm towel then soothing oils, such as peppermint, rosemary, or lavender, would be caressed into the feet to create a feeling of well-being. The Japanese used the ancient tradition of reflexology to promote health. It works on the basis that when a particular part of the foot is manipulated, stimulating energy will flow to a corresponding part of the body. The theraputic effects of this are felt throughout the body.

For the massage, create a minimalist space that is uncluttered and simple—a single flower in a vase, or a laquered tray for your oils. Dressed in a kimono you and your partner will feel elegant and relaxed. Several cushions will make your partner feel at ease as the massage will be given in a sitting position.

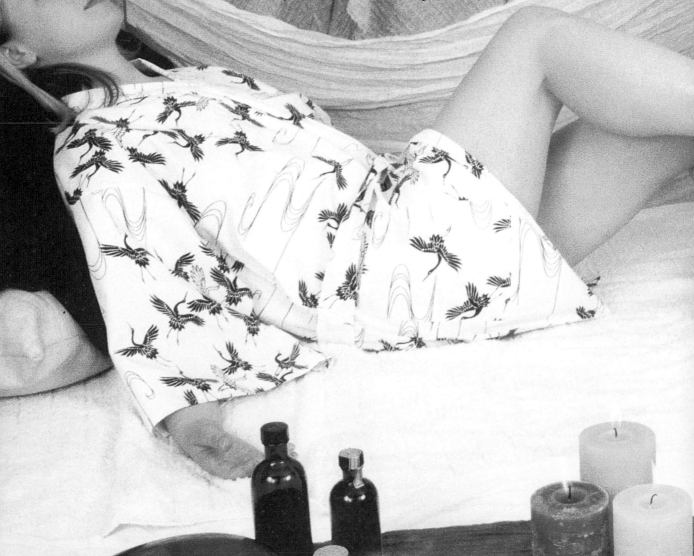

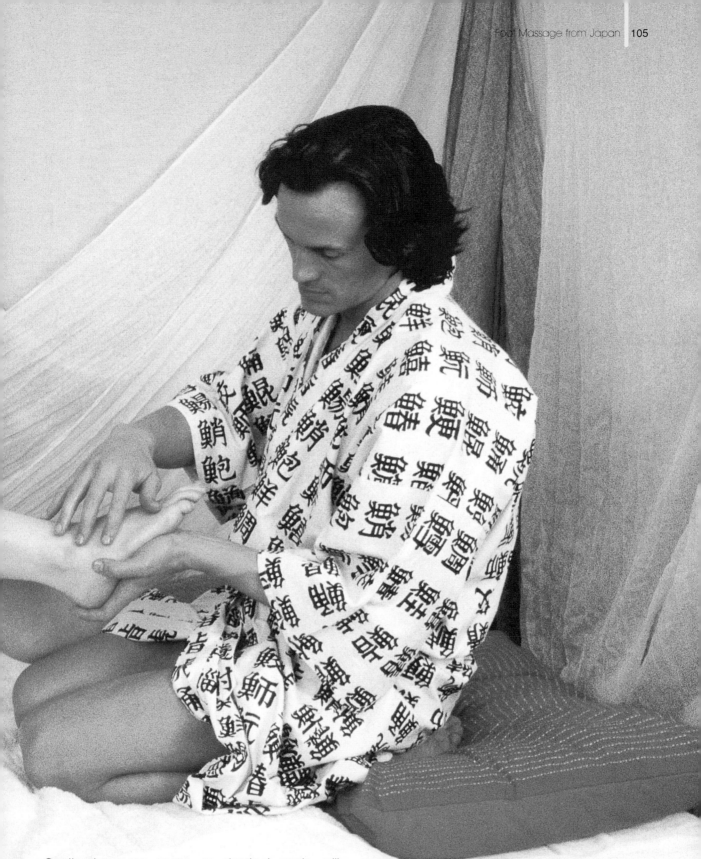

Gentle Japanese opera, or classical music, will complete the feeling of tranquillity and peace.

Choose a lightly perfumed soap and bathe or rinse the feet, using aromatic foot salts to ease any aches and pains. When everything is prepared and the room looks beautiful, invite your partner in and gently ease them into a restful position to pleasure the feet.

Bathing the Feet

Once in the sanctuary of their own homes the Japanese people are renowned for their rituals of cleansing and purification. On commencing your massage take time to wash your partner's feet and enjoy the all-over sensations that this will create.

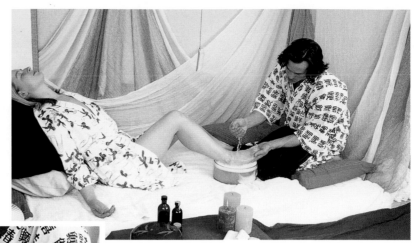

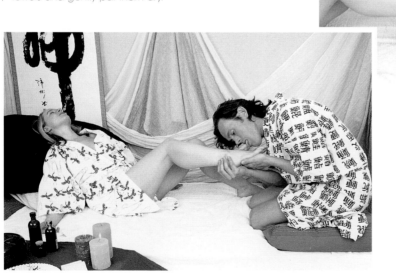

1 | Allow your partner to recline on soft pillows, and relax. Bend the knees and place the feet in a bowl of warm water. Gently lift one foot and start to wash it using slow, soothing movements. Leave the foot to soak in the warm water as you caress and wash the other one, then wrap them both in a soft, warm towel.

2 | Empty the bowl and refill it with clean, warm water, adding your herbal infusions or oils. Place your partner's feet in the bowl, and allow them to soak. Leave them to relax for 10–15 minutes. When your partner's feet have soaked thoroughly, wrap them tenderly in the warm, soft towels and gently pat them dry.

3 | When the feet are clean and dry, ask your partner to close their eyes, lean back and relax. Slowly pick up one foot and brush your hair, or a feather, over the skin of the foot. Sway from side to side, letting your hair slide over the foot, or drift the feather lightly in the same way.

4 | Now, starting from your partner's heel, lick the sole of the foot, over the top of the toes, finishing on the top of the foot. End at the ankle. The slight roughness of the tongue will send shivers of pleasure through their feet. Taking each toe in turn, gently kiss and suck them until they are all tingling, then blow on them to enhance the sensation.

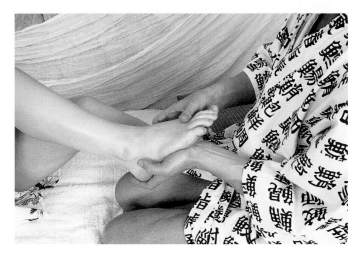

The Foot Massage

With their feet clean and revitalised your partner can now experience the pure delight of a full foot massage. Gentle sweeping strokes will send shivers from head to toe.

1 | Place your partner's foot on your knee then, having applied the oil, rest both hands on top of the foot, one in front of the other. Wrap your hands around the foot and glide them toward the ankle. When you reach the lower leg, separate and turn your hands so one hand is on the top of the leg and the other beneath. Squeeze your hands together and use firm strokes to massage the length of the foot.

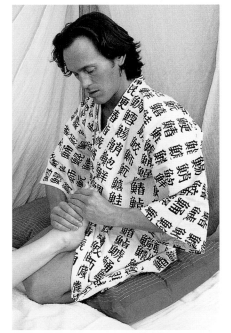

2 | Place both hands on top of the foot with the thumbs underneath. Using the wringing technique, rub your hands around the feet in opposite directions.

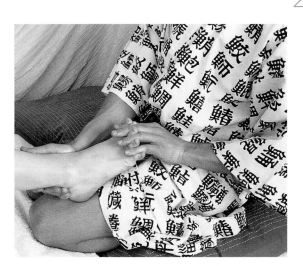

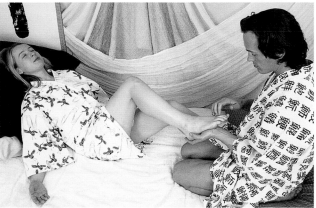

3 | Using one hand to hold the foot, cover the index finger of your other hand with oil and, very slowly, push, pull, and twist in between the toes, massaging the delicate valley areas. Use your fingers to massage between the toes, squeezing them, before drawing your fingers off the top.

4 | Using the pads of your fingers, brush them over the top of the foot from the ankle to the tip of the toes, one hand after the other, to tease and arouse the skin further. Repeat the stroke, but this time use your nails to make the skin tingle. To finish your massage, allow a few moments just to play with your partner's feet. Do whatever feels right, and whatever excites and thrills you both.

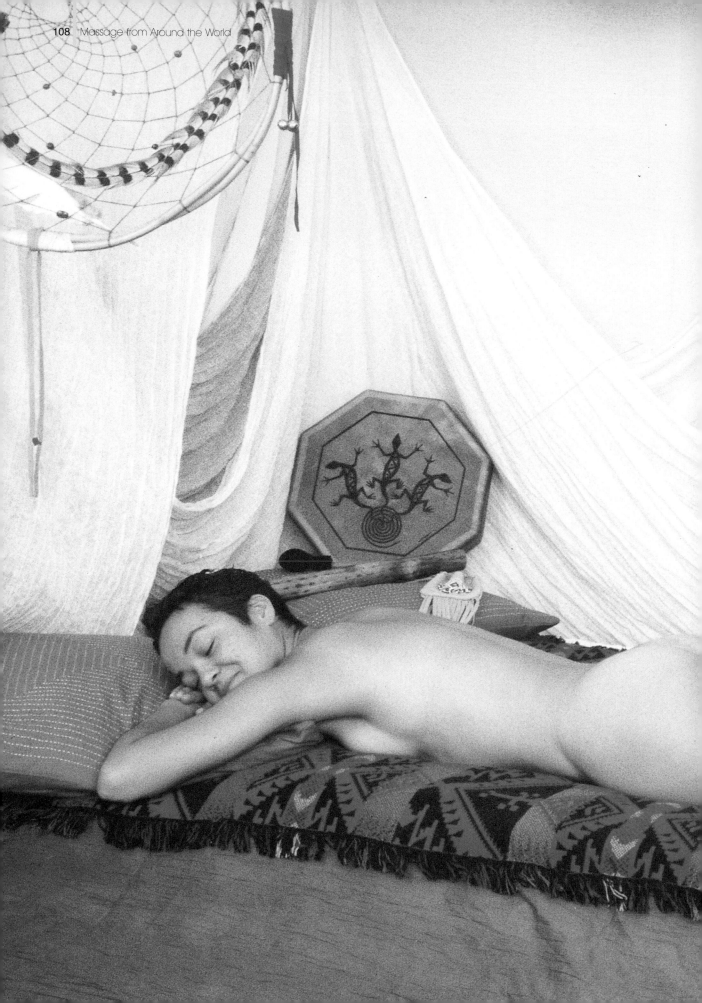

Rhythmic Massage from
Native America

The Native American Indians used the power of massage to awaken their inner spirits. They favored stimulating, vibrating percussion strokes to rouse and release the spirits. During acts of worship, the tribe would dance to the sensual pounding of the drums, swaying and moving to lose themselves completely in the music. The warm air would be fragranced with the aroma of rich, woody incenses from burning herbs, Before you begin, choose a room that is large enough for you to dance and massage in. Hang draping fabrics around the room and select the traditional colors of turquoise, coral, or beige. Place white feathers around the room as a sign of spirituality. Use a soft and luxurious sheepskin or a fleecy blanket to perform the massage on and make the air redolent with rich, sensual oils, such as sandalwood, juniper, pine, or cedarwood. Play tribal drum music, or Native American Indian chants. Light the room with pure beeswax candles or, for an added touch, position a dream-catcher, a talisman made from feathers and net, by the massage bed to catch bad dreams and release good ones.

Percussion Strokes

American Indians use firm strokes which dance quickly over the body. Using the percussion action, they alternate between light and strong movements keeping in rhythm with the music. The quick vibrating motion will stimulate blood flow, reviving tired limbs and awakening their muscles.

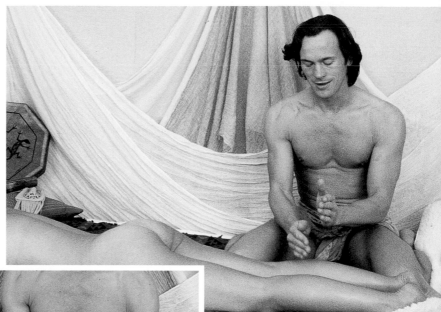

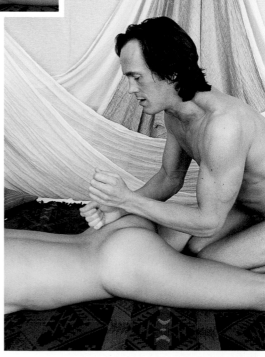

1 With your partner lying on the stomach, kneel beside the calves keeping your wrists nice and loose. Using the sides of your hands, in a prayer-like position, start to bounce them alternately on the calf. Keeping a steady rhythm, lightly and rapidly tap up and down the calf for about 20 seconds. Repeat on the other calf.

2 Now move on to the thighs and buttocks, repeating this percussion stroke over the whole area before again finishing with a slap. Move your position and repeat on the opposite leg. Gauge your partner's preferred pressure levels; too hard a movement will cause pain and discomfort, too soft and you will loose the energy of the stroke.

3 Kneeling between your partner's legs, use the sides of your hands and gently start to bounce your loose fists alternately over the sacrum. Begin quite slowly, then gradually let your rhythm grow faster, keeping a light, even pressure all over the lower back.

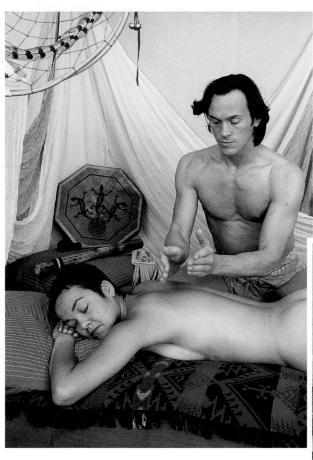

4 Move to your partner's upper back. Start with the percussion stroke up and down the back, then slow the movement down, working over the back and shoulders. Repeat this stroke either side of the spine.

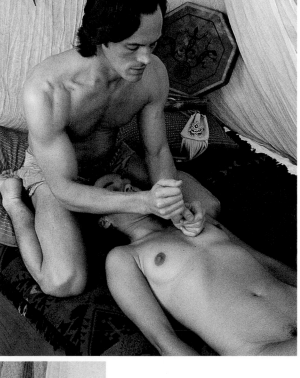

5 Turn your partner over and sit astride the head. Using your fists, start to gently and slowly massage your partner's upper chest and breast bone. When massaging a woman take particular care around the delicate breast area. Maintain the movement for about 60 seconds before finishing.

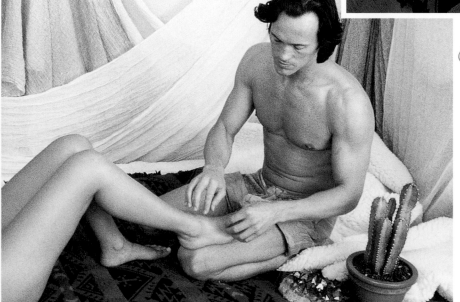

6 Let your partner take a few moments to feel the energy running through them. To finish, move down to your partner's feet and, with your fingertips, gently tap over one foot with the percussion stroke. This whole body massage is excellent for regeneration and can be repeated to leave the whole body tingling with pleasure.

Body Massage from China

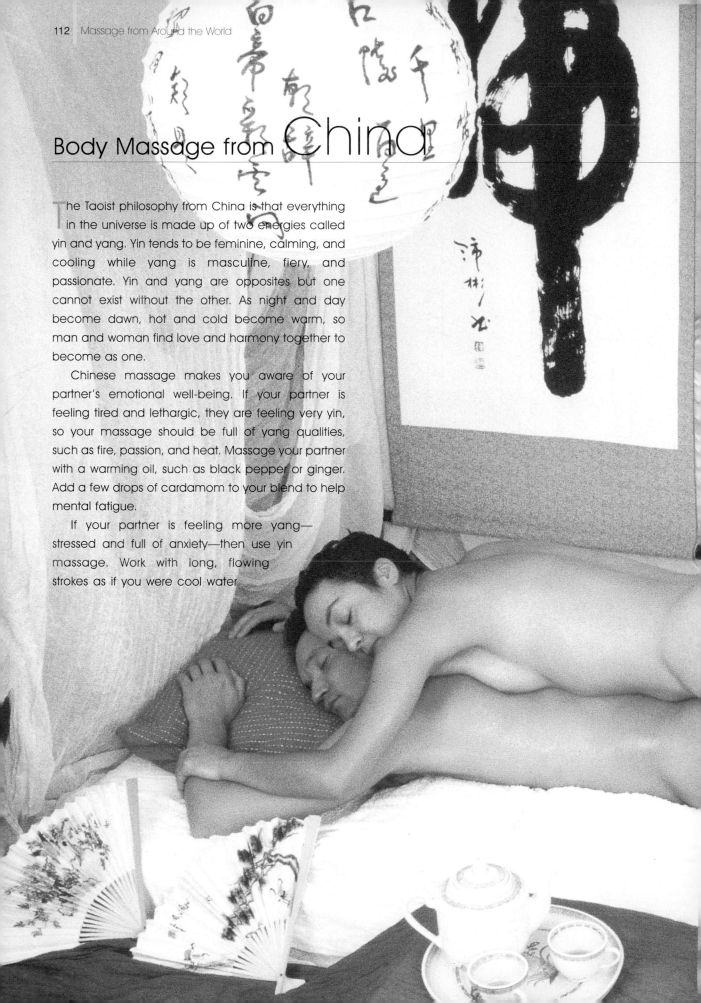

The Taoist philosophy from China is that everything in the universe is made up of two energies called yin and yang. Yin tends to be feminine, calming, and cooling while yang is masculine, fiery, and passionate. Yin and yang are opposites but one cannot exist without the other. As night and day become dawn, hot and cold become warm, so man and woman find love and harmony together to become as one.

Chinese massage makes you aware of your partner's emotional well-being. If your partner is feeling tired and lethargic, they are feeling very yin, so your massage should be full of yang qualities, such as fire, passion, and heat. Massage your partner with a warming oil, such as black pepper or ginger. Add a few drops of cardamom to your blend to help mental fatigue.

If your partner is feeling more yang—stressed and full of anxiety—then use yin massage. Work with long, flowing strokes as if you were cool water

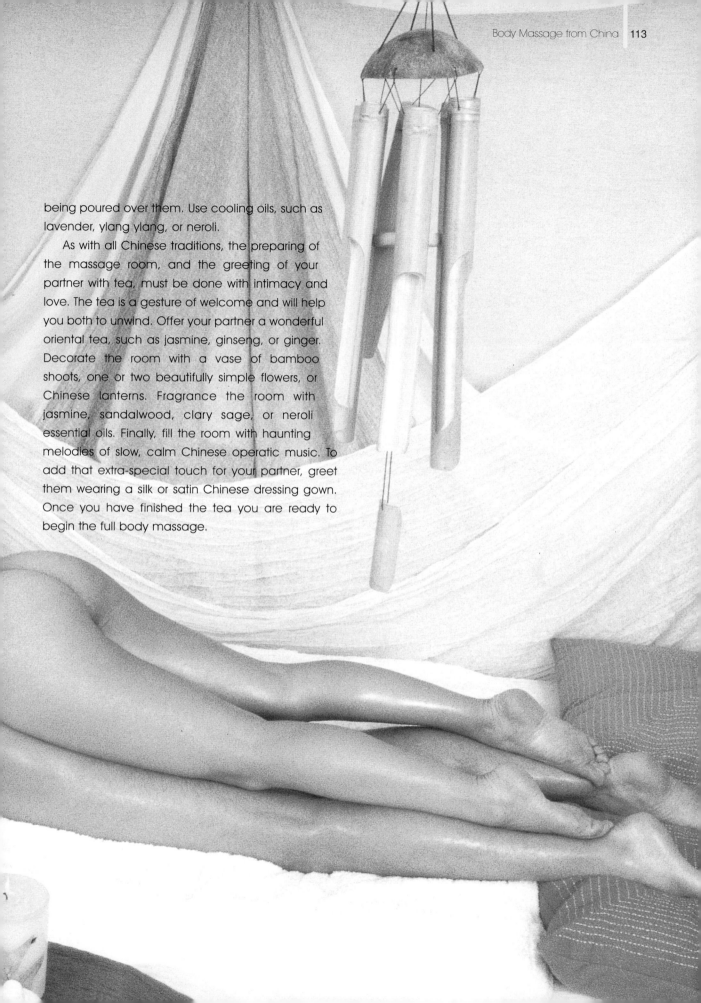

being poured over them. Use cooling oils, such as lavender, ylang ylang, or neroli.

As with all Chinese traditions, the preparing of the massage room, and the greeting of your partner with tea, must be done with intimacy and love. The tea is a gesture of welcome and will help you both to unwind. Offer your partner a wonderful oriental tea, such as jasmine, ginseng, or ginger. Decorate the room with a vase of bamboo shoots, one or two beautifully simple flowers, or Chinese lanterns. Fragrance the room with jasmine, sandalwood, clary sage, or neroli essential oils. Finally, fill the room with haunting melodies of slow, calm Chinese operatic music. To add that extra-special touch for your partner, greet them wearing a silk or satin Chinese dressing gown. Once you have finished the tea you are ready to begin the full body massage.

Body Massage

Chinese massage, using your whole body, is highly sensual and very arousing. You will need to generously anoint your body in a luxuriously fragranced oil for ease of movement.

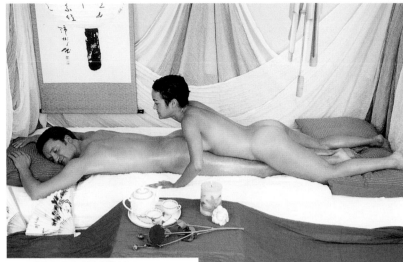

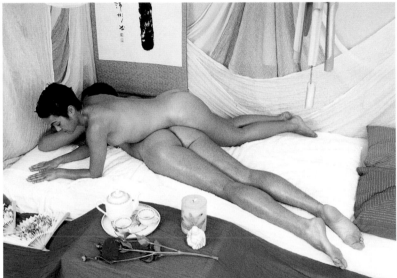

1 Lie your partner on their stomach, with arms stretched above the head. Kneel at their feet with your hands either side of their legs. Lower your chest against the soles of your partner's feet and, leaning some of your body weight on your hands, slowly slide up your partner's body. This will create a divine sensation.

2 When you are lying completely on top of your partner, gently lift your legs over theirs. Support your weight on your arms, and turn until you are lying across the back at 90°. Lean on your forearms, and caress the back and buttocks with your stomach.

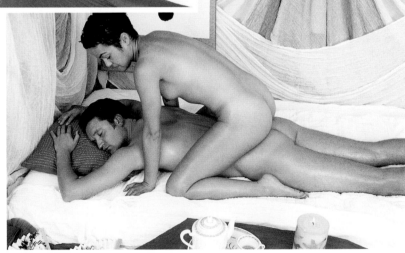

3 Glide back on top of your partner, and sit up and lean back so you are squatting over your partner's buttocks. Lean onto your hands and feet. Using the soft mounds of your buttocks, slide over your partner's buttocks, into the sensual curve of the back, and up the back, leaning most of your weight upon your hands and feet.

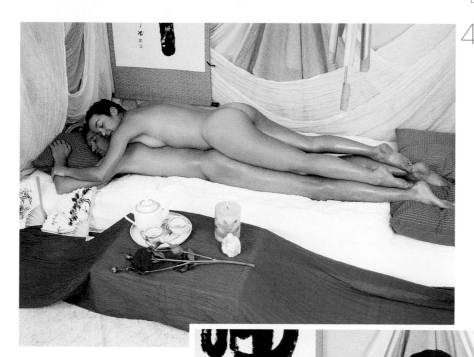

4 Lie across your partner with arms outstretched. Rest like this for a few moments as the two polarities of energy, yin and yang, become one between you. Turn your partner over, and repeat the slide. Rest your weight on the forearms if you are afraid of being too heavy.

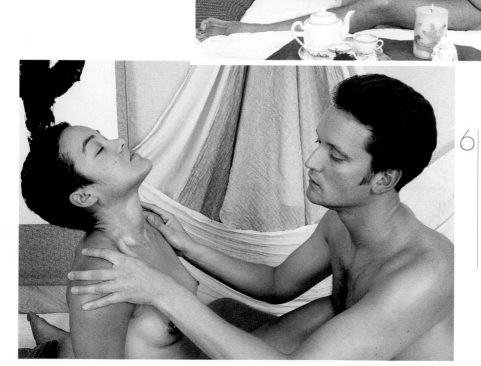

5 Another enjoyable way of embracing and massaging each other is to sit facing one another, with legs entwined. Start massaging over each other's backs with caressing, squeezing strokes or long, flowing stokes. Rest your head on each others shoulders,

6 Brush your hands over each other's stomachs and chests. Close your eyes and let your hands feel each other, and wrap your arms around one another. Drift gentle fingers over lips and eyes. Allow yourself to become one energy, creating a feeling of harmony and love.

CHAPTER 5
Sensual Treats

The therapeutic and healing effects of massage are well–known but you can also let your imagination run wild by using food in your massage, or turning it into a treat that you can offer as a gift.

Food is not only erotic, it can also be fun as the different sensations it creates can make you sigh deeply or laugh with joy. The different textures and temperatures of food can have a wonderful effect on the skin. The thick, syrup-like flow of honey with its sweet aroma contrasts well with the fluid, silky texture of fresh cream. Poured onto a

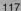

naked body they will make you shiver with delight. Food has often been associated with seduction in both literature and film, and its aphrodisiac properties go back for many thousands of years.

It is not surprising, therefore, that food should play an important part in sensual massage. The idea of licking food off a lover's body or drinking champagne in a bubble bath together is a treat few could refuse. As a special occasion you could use food in your massage for a partner's birthday or a celebration. Spend some time planning what you are going to use and make a gift out of the oils and candles that you place in the massage room. As well as spending time giving the massage it is important, once you have finished, to retain the closeness that a massage achieves. By lying together after the massage you can prolong the feeling of oneness, and share in the joy that comes from indulging in your partner.

Exotic foods of Love

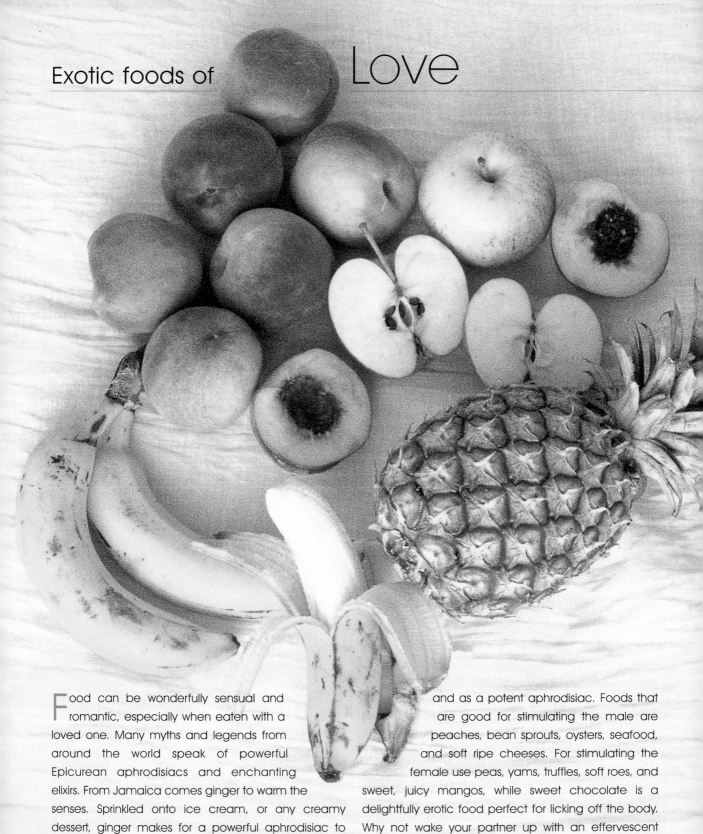

Food can be wonderfully sensual and romantic, especially when eaten with a loved one. Many myths and legends from around the world speak of powerful Epicurean aphrodisiacs and enchanting elixirs. From Jamaica comes ginger to warm the senses. Sprinkled onto ice cream, or any creamy dessert, ginger makes for a powerful aphrodisiac to spice up your love life. Medieval folklore used garlic in recipes to give stamina and vitality, to cleanse blood and as a potent aphrodisiac. Foods that are good for stimulating the male are peaches, bean sprouts, oysters, seafood, and soft ripe cheeses. For stimulating the female use peas, yams, truffles, soft roes, and sweet, juicy mangos, while sweet chocolate is a delightfully erotic food perfect for licking off the body. Why not wake your partner up with an effervescent champagne breakfast or treat them to a candlelit dinner in a special restaurant? Summer is a fantastic

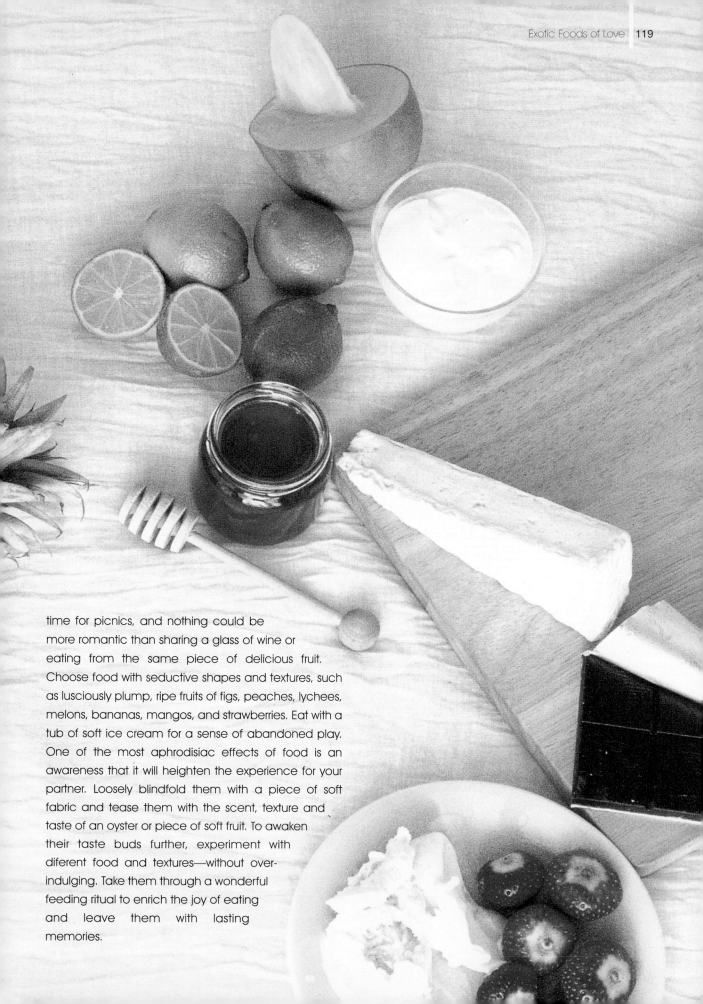

time for picnics, and nothing could be more romantic than sharing a glass of wine or eating from the same piece of delicious fruit. Choose food with seductive shapes and textures, such as lusciously plump, ripe fruits of figs, peaches, lychees, melons, bananas, mangos, and strawberries. Eat with a tub of soft ice cream for a sense of abandoned play. One of the most aphrodisiac effects of food is an awareness that it will heighten the experience for your partner. Loosely blindfold them with a piece of soft fabric and tease them with the scent, texture and taste of an oyster or piece of soft fruit. To awaken their taste buds further, experiment with diferent food and textures—without over-indulging. Take them through a wonderful feeding ritual to enrich the joy of eating and leave them with lasting memories.

A Birthday Surprise

Your partner's birthday draws near and you would like to treat them to a special birthday present but are completely lost for ideas. Why not treat them to a birthday massage?

Giving your partner a special birthday massage can be made even more memorable by lavishing all sorts of delicious treats on them, such as slowly trickling honey over their skin before lovingly licking it off. This is also a special way of showing your partner how much you love them.

Let your taste buds decide what food you would like to choose for the massage—cream, honey, ice cream, or even melted chocolate are ideal for this occasion. Use cream to slowly pour into your partner's navel, allowing it to gently overflow and trickle teasingly down the sides of the stomach, then move up the body, pouring as you go. Lick the

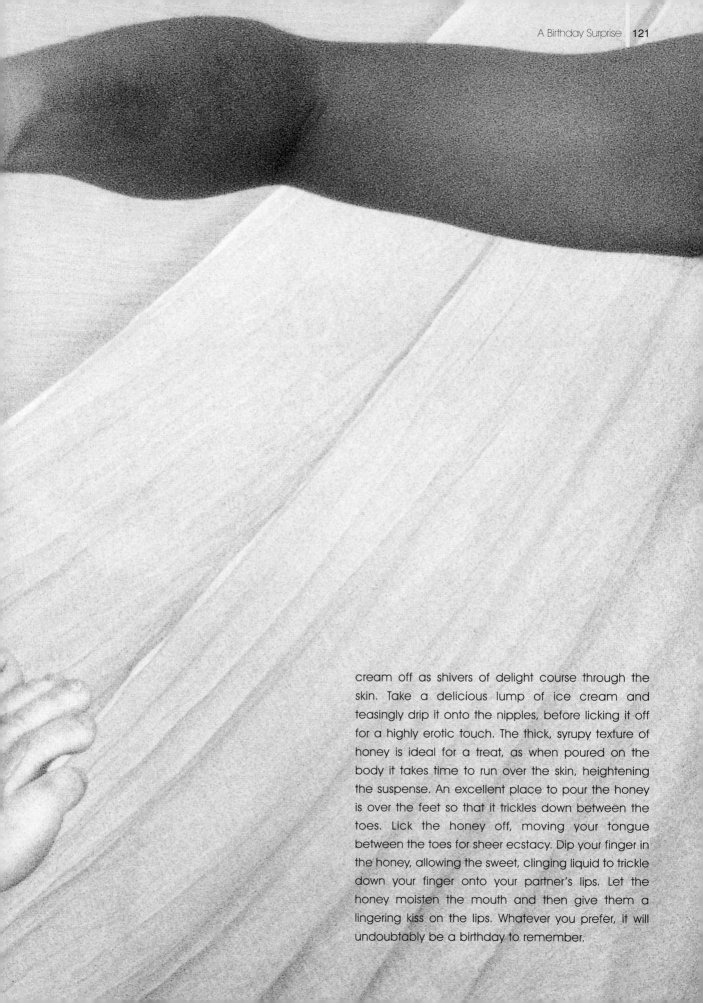

cream off as shivers of delight course through the skin. Take a delicious lump of ice cream and teasingly drip it onto the nipples, before licking it off for a highly erotic touch. The thick, syrupy texture of honey is ideal for a treat, as when poured on the body it takes time to run over the skin, heightening the suspense. An excellent place to pour the honey is over the feet so that it trickles down between the toes. Lick the honey off, moving your tongue between the toes for sheer ecstacy. Dip your finger in the honey, allowing the sweet, clinging liquid to trickle down your finger onto your partner's lips. Let the honey moisten the mouth and then give them a lingering kiss on the lips. Whatever you prefer, it will undoubtably be a birthday to remember.

Enjoying the Effects

Massage will bring both you and your partner many benefits, both physical and emotional. As well as stimulating blood flow, improving skin quality, and relaxing tense and tired muscles, it can be used every day to build intimacy in your relationship. You can take one or two sequences from Basic Sensual Strokes to give your partner a short massage after work, or use them as a special way of saying "thank you."

Massage also presents you with the perfect opportunity to set time aside for your partner; perhaps a quiet night in, when you can massage each other, and then spend the rest of the evening talking or holding one another. Or make the most of your weekends together by indulging in one of the soothing, sensual massages from around the world.

Special occasions can be made even more memorable by the introduction of massage. A day trip to the coast or a beach-side holiday can be enhanced by one of the meditative massages, such as the Indian chakra massage, which would serve as the perfect prelude to a gentle stroll on the beach. If you're planning an invigorating day's hiking, why not tune into nature with the Native Indian or Hawaiian massage? Alternatively, inject some excitement into your social life by preparing for a glamorous night out with the washing and shaving massages.

When you have finished massaging each other, and your bodies feel light and are tingling with pleasure, you will find that you have awoken new

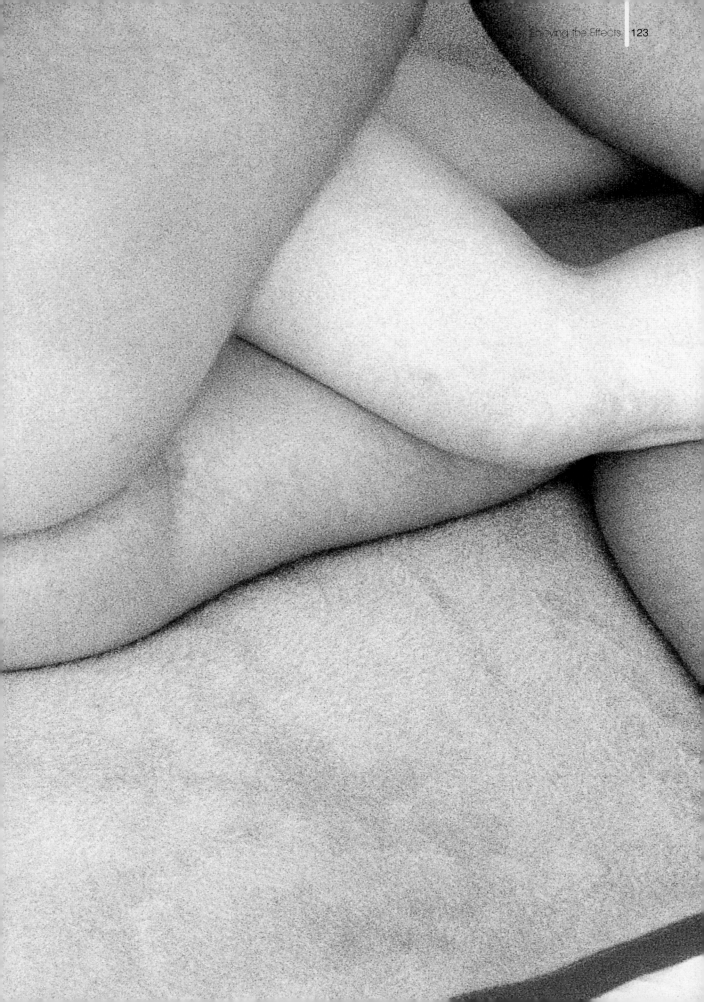

feelings of tenderness and sensuality in each other. These wonderful sensations do not always have to lead to sexual play—you can simply luxuriate in the feelings of warmth and intimacy that your massage has induced. If you wish to achieve further feelings of well-being, or even sleep, treat your partner to a soothing massage, and then gently cuddle up alongside them, and cover yourselves with a soft, warm blanket. Wrap your arms around your partner to provide them with a reassuring feeling of being safe and loved. Remain like this for as long as you please, for you may also find that massage brings with it wonderful sleep.

Massage gives you and your partner the chance to relish the blissful luxury of being together, away from the stresses of everyday life and you don't need to be a sexual athlete to enjoy it. Never underestimate the importance of affection, and the pleasure that being touched and held can bring. View massage as a romantic gift that you can give your partner, something more than chocolates!

We have demonstrated massage in different settings, for different occasions, and with different oil recipes. Remember above all, to use your imagination and adapt our ideas and suggestions to what you and your partner enjoy most.

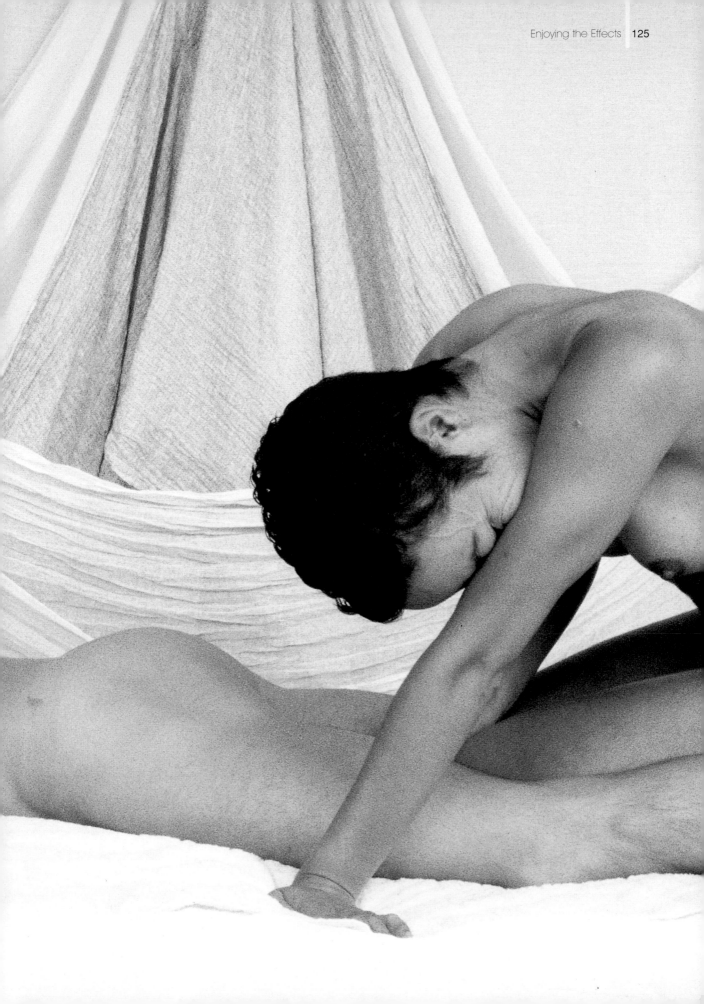

Index

AUTHOR'S ACKNOWLEDGEMENTS

I would like to thank Meghan Tilson for her hard work and patience in helping me edit and type up my writing for the book.

THE MODELS
Who made the hardwork of the photo sessions great fun and a pleasure to do:
Geoff Burton, Robert Clarke, Eleana Barquilla, Pauline Hau, Naomi Depeza and Andrea Cameron-Cooper

Will White, the photographer, for his exquisite photographs and great sense of humor.

Francis Cawley and Joyce Bentley for their hard work at Quarto.

Finally I would like to thank my two greatest massage teachers, Fiona Harrold and Isabel Hughes.

For further courses on massage, please contact:

The London College of Massage
5 Newman Passage
London W1P 3PF

Tel: 0171 323 3574

SPECIAL THANKS TO:

Neal Street East, 7 Neal Street, Covent Garden, London, for the loan of items featured in the 'Massage Around the World' section.